15,000+
Baby
Names

Bruce Lansky

Meadowbrook Press

Distributed by Simon & Schuster
New York

Acknowledgments

"Guidelines For Naming Your Baby" was excerpted from *The Best Baby Name Book In The Whole Wide World,* © 1984 by Bruce Lansky, reprinted with permission of Meadowbrook, Inc.

The lists of the 100 most popular boys' and girls' names were compiled by Michael Clingman at the Social Security Administration.

"The Baby Name List" was excerpted in abridged form from *35,000 Baby Names* © 1995 by Bruce Lansky, reprinted with permission of Meadowbrook Press.

Library of Congress Cataloging In Publication Data
Lansky, Bruce.
    15,000 baby names / Bruce Lansky.
       p.   cm.
    ISBN 0-88166-282-8 (Meadowbrook)
    ISBN 0-671-52127-6 (Simon & Schuster)
    1. Names, Personal—Dictionaries. I. Title.
  CS2377.L345 1997
  929.4'4'03—dc21   97-7031
                                  CIP

© 1997 by Bruce Lansky

Published by Meadowbrook Press, 5451 Smetana Drive, Minnetonka, MN 55343

www.meadowbrookpress.com

Book trade distribution by Simon & Schuster, a division of Simon and Schuster, Inc. 1230 Avenue of the Americas, New York, New York 10020

06 05 04   20 19 18 17 16 15

Printed in the United States of America

Editor: Liya Lev Oertel
Production Manager: Joe Gagne
Production Assistant: Danielle White
Cover Photography: Peter PoonOnWong

Contents

15,000+
Baby
Names

The Most Popular
Names In the
United States

The popularity of names, like the length of hemlines and the width of ties, is subject to change every year. The changes become even more noticeable when you think about the changes in name "fashions" over longer periods.

Think about the names of your grandparents and famous entertainers of their generation: Bette Davis, Dorothy Lamour, Rhonda Flemming, Helen Hayes, Margaret O'Brien, Ralph Bellamy, Fred Astaire, Gary Cooper, Frank Sinatra—none of their first names is in the current list of top 100 names.

Popular entertainers of the 1950s included Debbie Reynolds, Doris Day, Rock Hudson, and Patti Page—none of their first names is in the current list of top 100 names either.

It seems that in every decade a new group of names rises in popularity, as names associated with a previous generation of babies decline. So, it is wise to consider whether a name's popularity is rising, declining, or holding steady.

To help you assess name popularity trends, we are presenting the top 100 names given to baby boys and girls during the past year. The rankings are derived from a survey of new birth records nationwide, conducted by the Social Security Administration.

As you refer to the following data, remember that the popularity issue cuts two ways: 1) Psychologists say a child with a common or popular name seems to have better odds of success in life than a child with an uncommon name. 2) A child whose name is at the top of the popularity poll may not feel as unique and special as a child whose name is less common.

The Top 100 Girls' Names in 2001

1. Emily
2. Hannah
3. Madison
4. Samantha
5. Ashley
6. Sarah
7. Elizabeth
8. Kayla
9. Alexis
10. Abigail
11. Jessica
12. Taylor
13. Anna
14. Lauren
15. Megan
16. Brianna
17. Olivia
18. Victoria
19. Emma
20. Grace
21. Rachel
22. Jasmine
23. Nicole
24. Destiny
25. Alyssa
26. Chloe
27. Julia
28. Jennifer
29. Kaitlyn
30. Morgan
31. Isabella
32. Natalie
33. Alexandra
34. Sydney
35. Katherine
36. Amanda
37. Stephanie
38. Hailey
39. Maria
40. Gabrielle
41. Haley
42. Rebecca
43. Madeline
44. Sophia
45. Mary
46. Amber
47. Courtney
48. Jenna
49. Jordan
50. Sierra
51. Bailey
52. Mackenzie
53. Gabriella
54. Sara
55. Jada
56. Katelyn
57. Savannah
58. Kaylee
59. Allison
60. Andrea
61. Catherine
62. Danielle
63. Zoe
64. Alexa
65. Christina
66. Ariana
67. Caitlin
68. Michelle
69. Brooke
70. Kimberly
71. Makayla
72. Shelby
73. Trinity
74. Erin
75. Jade
76. Mariah
77. Melanie
78. Alexandria
79. Angela
80. Arianna
81. Jacqueline
82. Paige
83. Faith
84. Melissa
85. Riley
86. Vanessa
87. Ana
88. Isabel
89. Isabelle
90. Kelly
91. Marissa
92. Alexia
93. Angelica
94. Brittany
95. Jocelyn
96. Miranda
97. Mya
98. Caroline
99. Cassidy
100. Jordyn

The Top 100 Boys' Names in 2001

1. Jacob	35. Thomas	69. Jared
2. Michael	36. Kyle	70. Bryan
3. Joshua	37. Kevin	71. Garrett
4. Matthew	38. Gabriel	72. Steven
5. Andrew	39. Elijah	73. Adrian
6. Joseph	40. Jason	74. Cody
7. Nicholas	41. Luis	75. Charles
8. Anthony	42. Aaron	76. Devin
9. Tyler	43. Caleb	77. Eduardo
10. Daniel	44. Connor	78. Richard
11. Christopher	45. Luke	79. Marcus
12. Alexander	46. Jordan	80. Ian
13. John	47. Jack	81. Lucas
14. William	48. Adam	82. Seth
15. Brandon	49. Eric	83. Xavier
16. Dylan	50. Jackson	84. Dalton
17. Zachary	51. Carlos	85. Jeremiah
18. Ethan	52. Angel	86. Miguel
19. Ryan	53. Isaiah	87. Blake
20. Justin	54. Alex	88. Edward
21. David	55. Evan	89. Wyatt
22. Benjamin	56. Mason	90. Fernando
23. Christian	57. Isaac	91. Spencer
24. Austin	58. Jesus	92. Antonio
25. Cameron	59. Sean	93. Carson
26. James	60. Timothy	94. Gavin
27. Jonathan	61. Patrick	95. Julian
28. Logan	62. Brian	96. Oscar
29. Nathan	63. Bryce	97. Trevor
30. Samuel	64. Nathaniel	98. Tristan
31. Hunter	65. Chase	99. Aidan
32. Noah	66. Juan	100. Dakota
33. Robert	67. Sebastian	
34. Jose	68. Cole	

Guidelines For
Naming Your Baby
15 Things to Consider

1. Namesakes

Exact reproductions of a parent's name, even if it is followed by Jr. or II, are often confusing to everyone involved. Parents frequently vary the middle name of a son who carries his father's first and last names, and then call the son by his middle name to distinguish him from his father; but the potential for confusion still exists. What's worse, the child never gets the satisfaction of having a name and a clear identity of his own.

Namesakes can lead to unhappy choices of names for the child, too. Somehow the name Mildred just doesn't seem to fit a little girl comfortably, even though it fits 80-year-old Aunt Mildred perfectly. Generally, it's wiser to be certain a namesake's name is one you'd choose on its own merits, quite apart from the good feelings you have for the person you're complimenting this way.

2. Nationality

If you choose a "foreign-sounding" name, be sure it's not unpronounceable or unspellable, or the name will be a burden to your child. Combinations of names from different countries, like Francoise Finklebaum or Marco Mazarowski, may provoke smiles. So if you want to combine names with different ethnic roots, try them out on lots of people before making a final decision.

3. Religion

To some parents it is important to follow religious traditions in naming a baby. Roman Catholics have traditionally chosen saints' names, sometimes using Mary as a first name for each daughter and pairing it with different middle names: Mary Rose, Mary Margaret, and so on. Jews traditionally choose Old Testament names, often the name of a deceased relative, while Protestants choose both Old and New Testament names. Muslims turn to the Koran and the names of Mohammed and his family as traditional sources of names

4. Gender

There are two opposing lines of thought on names that can be given to boys and girls alike, whether they are changeable ones like Carol/Caroll, Leslie/Lesley, and Claire/ Clair or the truly unisex names like Robin, Chris, and Terry. Some parents feel that a unisex name allows them to pick it with certainty before the baby's sex is known and that such names "type" children in sexual roles and expectations less than traditional boy-girl names do. Others argue that it's unfair and psychologically harmful to require a child to explain which sex he or she is (remember the song, "A Boy Named Sue"?). Finally, boys feel more threatened or insulted when they are presumed to be girls then girls do when they're taken to be boys.

5. Number of Names

No law requires a person to have three names, though most forms provide spaces for a first name, middle initial or name and surname. When choosing a name for your child, you have several options: a first and last name; a first and last name and only a middle initial (Harry S Truman's S is just an S); initials for both first and middle names; or several middle names. Keep your child's lifelong use of the name in mind when you do something unusual—four middle names are going to cause space problems for your child every time he or she fills out a form!

6. Sounds

The combination of letters in a person's name can make saying the name easier or harder. Alliteration, as in Tina Turner or Pat Paulsen, is fine, but such rhymes as Tyrone Cohn or Alice Palace invite teasing. Joke names, punning names, and other displays of wit may sound funny, but living with such a name is no laughing matter.

7. Rhythms

Most naming specialists agree that unequal numbers of syllables create pleasing rhythms. Such names as Dwight David Eisenhower or Molly Melinda Grooms fit this pattern. When first and last names have equal numbers of syllables, a middle name with a different number creates a nice effect, as in

Albert Anthony Cleveland or Gail Canova Pons. Single-sylla-
ble names can be especially forceful if each name has a rather
long sound, as in Mark Twain or Charles Rath.

8. Pronunciation

Nobody likes having their name constantly mispronounced.
If you pick an unusual name, such as Jésus or Genviéve (Hay-
soos and Zhan-vee-ev), don't expect people to pronounce it
correctly. Other names with high mispronunciation potential
are names that have more than one common pronunciation,
as in Alicia (does the second syllable rhyme with fish or
leash?) or Shana (does the name rhyme with Anna or Dana?).
And if you choose a unique pronunciation for a name (for
example pronouncing Nina like Dinah), don't expect many
people to get it right.

9. Spelling

In his poem *Don Juan,* Byron writes, "Thrice happy is he
whose name has been well spelt," and it's true that you feel a
special kind of irritation when your name gets misspelled.
   Ordinary spellings have the force of common sense
behind them. On the other hand, a new or unusual spelling
can revitalize an old name. If the name Ethel only reminds
you of Ether Mertz in the old *I Love Lucy* show, but your mate
is crazy about having a daughter with that name, perhaps
Ethelle will be a happy substitute. However, some people
think it's silly to vary from "traditional" spelling of names and
are prejudiced against any Thom, Dik, or Hari.

10. Popularity

Some names are so popular you shouldn't be surprised to find
more than one child with that name in your child's classroom.
A child with a very popular name may feel that he or she must
"share" it with others, while a child with a very uncommon
name is likely to feel that it is uniquely his or hers. However, a
child with a popular name may be accepted by peers more
easily than a child with a very uncommon name, which may
be perceived as weird.

11. Uniqueness

Did you ever try to look in the phone book for the telephone number of someone called John Smith? You wouldn't be able to find it without also knowing the address. To avoid confusion, many people with common last names choose distinctive first and/or middle names for their children. However, a highly unusual name, such as Teague or Hestia, could be an even greater disservice to your child than Michael or Emily.

12. Stereotypes

Most names call to mind physical or personality traits that often stem from a well-known namesake, real or fictional. Some names—Adolph and Judas, for instance—may never outlive the terrible associations they receive from a single person who bore them. Because the image of a name will affect its owner's self-image, as well as the way he or she is perceived by others, consider what associations come to mind as you make your selections.

13. Initials

Folk wisdom has it that a person whose initials spell a word—any word—is destined to be successful in life. But it can be irksome, even embarrassing, to have DUD or HAG stamped on your suitcases and jewelry. So be sure your child's initials spell "happy" words—or none at all—to avoid these problems.

14. Nicknames

Most names have shortened or familiar forms that are used during childhood or at different stages of life. For example, Michael might be called Mikey as a child, Mike as a teenager, and Michael on his college application. So, if you don't want your daughter called Sam, don't name her Samantha.

If you're thinking of giving your child a nickname as a legal name, remember that Trisha may grow weary of explaining that her real name is not Patricia. And consider the fact that names that sound cute for a child, as in Missy and Timmy, could prove embarrassing later in life. Can you picture Grandma Missy and Grandpa Timmy?

15. Meanings

Most people don't know the meanings of their names—first, middle, or last. But most names do have meanings, and you should at least find out what your favorite choices mean before giving them to your child. A name that means something funny or embarrassing probably won't overshadow your child's life, but if you have to choose between two names that are equally attractive to you, meanings may help tip the balance.

Girls' Names

Abbey, Abbie, Abby
(Hebrew) familiar forms
of Abigail.
Abbe, Abbi, Abbye, Abia

Abigail (Hebrew) father's
joy. Bible: one of the wives
of King David. See also
Gail.
**Abagael, Abagail,
Abagale, Abagil,
Abbegail, Abbegale,
Abbegayle, Abbey,
Abbigail, Abbigale,
Abbigayle, Abbygail,
Abbygale, Abbygayle,
Abegail, Abegale,
Abegayle, Abgail, Abgale,
Abgayle, Abigael, Abigal,
Abigale, Abigayil,
Abigayle, Abigel, Avigail**

Ada (German) a short
form of Adelaide.
(English) prosperous;
happy.
**Adabelle, Adah, Adalee,
Adan, Adda, Addia,
Addie, Adia, Adiah, Auda,
Aude**

Addie (Greek, German)
a familiar form of Adelaide,
Adrienne.

**Adde, Addey, Addi, Addia,
Addy, Adey, Adi, Adie,
Ady, Atti, Attie, Atty**

Adelaide (German) noble
and serene. See also Ada,
Adeline, Adele, Delia,
Della, Heidi.
**Adeela, Adelade, Adelaid,
Adelaida, Adelei,
Adelheid, Adeliade,
Adelka, Aley, Laidey, Laidy**

Adele (German, English)
a short form of Adelaide,
Adeline.
**Adel, Adela, Adelia,
Adelista, Adell, Adella,
Adelle**

Adeline (English) a form of
Adelaide.
**Adalina, Adaline, Addie,
Adelina, Adelind, Adelita,
Adeliya, Adelle, Adelyn,
Adelynn, Adena, Adilene,
Adina, Adinna, Adlena,
Adlene, Adlin, Adline,
Aline, Alita**

Adina (Hebrew) noble;
adorned. See also Dina.
**Adiana, Adiena, Adinah,
Adinna**

Adriana, Adrianna
(Italian) forms of Adrienne.
Adrea, Adria

Adriane, Adrianne
(English) forms of
Adrienne.

Adrienne (Greek) rich.
(Latin) dark. A feminine
form of Adrian.

Adrienne *(cont.)*
Addie, Adrien, Adriana,
Adriane, Adrianna,
Adrianne, Adrie, Adrien,
Adriena, Adrienna

Afton (English) from Afton,
England.
Aftan, Aftine, Aftyn

Agatha (Greek) good,
kind. Literature: Agatha
Christie was a British
writer of more than
seventy detective novels.
Agace, Agasha, Agata,
Agathe, Agathi, Agatka,
Aggie, Ágota, Ágotha,
Agueda, Atka

Agnes (Greek) pure.
See also Anisha.
Aganetha, Aggie,
Agna, Agne, Agneis,
Agnelia, Agnella, Agnés,
Agnesa, Agnesca,
Agnese, Agnesina,
Agness, Agnesse,
Agneta, Agneti, Agnetta,
Agnies, Agnieszka,
Agniya, Agnola, Aignéis,
Aneska, Anka, Inez, Nessa

Aileen (Scottish) light
bearer. (Irish) a form of
Helen. See also Eileen.
Ailean, Ailene, Aili, Ailina,
Ailinn, Aleen, Aleena,
Aleene, Alene, Aliana,
Alianna, Alina, Aline,
Allene, Alline, Allyn,
Alyna, Alyne, Alynne

Aimee (Latin) an alternate
form of Amy. (French)
loved.
Aime, Aimée, Aimey,
Aimi, Aimia, Aimie, Aimy

Ainsley (Scottish) my own
meadow.
Ainslee, Ainsleigh, Ainslie,
Ainsly, Ansley, Aynslee,
Aynsley, Aynslie

Aisha (Swahili) life. (Arabic)
woman. See also Asha,
Asia, Iesha, Keisha.
Aesha, Aeshah, Aiesha,
Aieshah, Aishah, Aishia,
Aishiah, Ayasha, Ayesha,
Ayeshah, Ayisha, Ayishah,
Aysa, Ayse, Aysha,
Ayshah, Ayshe, Ayshea,
Aytza, Azia

Aja (Hindi) goat.
Ajah, Ajaran, Ajha, Ajia

Alaina, Alayna (Irish)
alternate forms of Alana.
Alaine, Alainna, Alainnah,
Alane, Alayne, Aleine,
Alleyna, Alleynah, Alleyne

Alana (Irish) attractive;
peaceful. (Hawaiian) offer-
ing. A feminine form of
Alan. See also Lana.
Alaina, Alanah, Alani,
Alania, Alanis, Alanna,
Alannah, Alawna, Alayna,
Allana, Allanah, Allyn

Alea, Aleah (Arabic) high,
exalted. (Persian) God's
being.

**Aleea, Aleeah, Alia,
Alleea, Alleeah, Allia**

Alecia (Greek) a form
of Alicia.
Alecea, Alesha

Alejandra (Spanish) a form
of Alexandra.
**Alejanda, Alejandr,
Alejandrea, Alejandria,
Alejandrina**

Alena (Russian) a form
of Helen.
**Aleen, Aleena, Alenah,
Alene, Alenka, Allene,
Alyna**

Alesha (Greek) an alternate
form of Alecia, Alisha.
**Aleasha, Aleashea, Aleasia,
Aleesha, Aleeshah,
Aleeshia, Aleeshya,
Aleisha, Aleshia, Alesia**

Alessandra (Italian) a form
of Alexandra.
**Alesandra, Alesandrea,
Allesand, Allesia, Allessa**

Alex, Alexa (Greek) short
forms of Alexandra.
Alekia, Aleksa, Aleksha

Alexandra (Greek)
defender of mankind.
A feminine form of
Alexander. History: the last
czarina of Russia. See also
Sandra, Sasha, Sondra.
**Alandra, Aleix, Alejandra,
Aleka, Aleks, Aleksandra,
Aleksasha, Alessandra,
Alexande, Alexina,**

**Alexine, Alexis, Alexx,
Alexxandra, Alexzand,
Alexzandra, Ali, Alix,
Aljexi, Alla, Lexandra**

Alexandria (Greek) an
alternate form of
Alexandra.
**Alexanderia, Alexanderina,
Alexanderine, Alexandrea,
Alexandrena, Alexandrie,
Alexandrina, Alexandrine,
Alexia, Alexzandrea,
Alexzandria**

Alexia (Greek) a short form
of Alexandria.
**Aleksey, Aleksi, Aleska,
Alexey, Alexi, Alexie, Alka,
Alya**

Alexis (Greek) a short form
of Alexandra.
**Alexcis, Alexes, Alexi,
Alexiou, Alexisia, Alexius,
Alexsia, Alexus, Alexx,
Alexxis, Alexys, Alexyss,
Lexis**

Ali (Greek) a familiar form
of Alicia, Alisha, Alison.
Allea, Alli, Allie, Ally, Aly

Alia (Hebrew) an alternate
form of Aliya. See also
Alea.
Aleana, Aliyah, Alya

Alice (Greek) truthful.
(German) noble. See also
Alisa, Alison, Allie, Alycia,
Alysa, Alyssa, Alysse.
**Adelice, Ailis, Alecia,
Aleece, Alica, Alican,
Alicie, Alicyn, Aliece,**

Alice *(cont.)*
**Alies, Aliese, Alika, Alis,
Alison, Alix, Alize, Alla,
Alleece, Alles, Allesse,
Allice, Allie, Allis, Allisa,
Allise, Allisse, Allix**

Alicia (English) an alternate
form of Alice. See also
Elicia.
**Alecia, Aleecia, Ali,
Alicea, Alicha, Alichia,
Alician, Alicja, Alicya,
Aliecia, Alisha, Allicea,
Alycia, Ilysa**

Alida (Latin) small and
winged. (Spanish) noble.
**Aleda, Aleta, Alidia, Alita,
Alleda, Allida, Allidah,
Alyda, Alydia, Elida**

Alina, Aline (Slavic)
bright. (Scottish) fair.
(English) a short form of
Adeline. See also Alena.
**Allene, Allyna, Allyne,
Alyna, Alyne**

Alisa, Alissa (Greek) an
alternate form of Alice.
See also Elisa.
**Alisia, Alise, Alisse, Alisza,
Alisse, Alisza, Alyssa**

Alisha (Greek) truthful.
(German) noble. (English)
an alternate form of Alicia.
See also Elisha.
**Aleesha, Alesha, Ali,
Aliesha, Alieshai, Aliscia,
Alishah, Alishay, Alishaye,
Alishea, Alishya, Alisia,
Alissia, Alitsha, Alysha**

Alison, Allison (English)
a form of Alice.
**Ali, Alicen, Alicyn,
Alisann, Alisanne, Alisen,
Alisson, Alisun, Alisyn,
Alles, Allesse, Allie, Allis,
Allise, Allix, Allsun**

Alix (Greek) a short form
of Alexandra, Alice.
Allix, Alyx

Aliya (Hebrew) ascender.
**Alea, Aleah, Alee, Aleea,
Aleia, Aleya, Alia, Aliyah,
Aly**

Aliza (Hebrew) joyful.
See also Eliza.
**Aleeza, Alieza, Aliezah,
Alitza, Alizah**

Allie (Greek) a familiar form
of Alice.
**Ali, Aleni, Alenna, Alleen,
Allene, Alline**

Allyson, Alyson (English)
alternate forms of Alison,
Allison.
**Allysen, Allyson, Allysun,
Alyson**

Alma (Arabic) learned.
(Latin) soul.
Almah

Alycia (English) an alternate form of Alicia.
Allyce, Alycea, Lycia, Alyse

Alysa, Alyse, Alysse
(Greek) alternate forms
of Alice.
**Allys, Allyse, Allyss, Alys,
Alyss**

Alysha, Alysia (Greek) alternate forms of Alisha.
Allysea, Allyscia, Alysea, Alyshia, Alyssha, Alyssia

Alyssa (Greek) rational. Botany: alyssum is a flowering herb. See also Alice, Elissa.
Alissa, Allissa, Allyssa, Ilyssa, Lyssa, Lyssah

Alysse (Greek) an alternate form of Alice.
Allyce, Allys, Allyse, Allyss, Alys, Alyss

Amanda (Latin) lovable.
Amada, Amanada, Amandah, Amandalee, Amandalyn, Amandi, Amandie, Amandine, Amandy

Amaris (Hebrew) promised by God.
Amarissa, Maris

Amber (French) amber.
Amberia, Amberise, Amberly, Ambur

Amelia (Latin) an alternate form of Emily. (German) hardworking. History: Amelia Earhart, an American aviator, was the first woman to fly solo across the Atlantic Ocean.
Amalia, Amaliya, Ameila, Ameley, Amelie, Amélie, Amelina, Ameline, Amelisa, Amelita, Amella, Amilia, Amilina, Amilisa, Amilita, Amillia, Amilyn, Amylia

Amelie (German) a familiar form of Amelia.
Amaley, Amalie, Amelee

Amina (Arabic) trustworthy, faithful. History: the mother of the prophet Mohammed.
Aminah, Aminda, Amindah, Aminta, Amintah

Amy (Latin) beloved. See also Aimee, Emma.
Amata, Ame, Amey, Ami, Amia, Amie, Amiet, Amii, Amiiee, Amijo, Amiko, Amio, Ammie, Ammy, Amye, Amylyn

Ana (Hawaiian, Spanish) a form of Hannah.
Anabela

Anais (Hebrew) gracious.
Anaise, Anaïse

Anastasia (Greek) resurrection. See also Stacey, Stacia.
Ana, Anastace, Anastacia, Anastacie, Anastase, Anastasha, Anastashia, Anastasie, Anastassia, Anastassya, Anastatia, Anastazia, Anastice, Annstás, Nastasia

Andrea (Greek) strong; courageous. (Latin) feminine. A feminine form of Andrew.

Andrea *(cont.)*
Aindrea, Andee, Andera,
Anderea, Andra, Andrah,
Andraia, Andraya,
Andreah, Andreaka,
Andrean, Andreana,
Andreane, Andreanna,
Andreanne, Andree,
Andrée, Andreea,
Andreia, Andreja,
Andreka, Andrel, Andrell,
Andrelle, Andrena,
Andrene, Andreo,
Andressa, Andrette,
Andrewina, Andreya,
Andri, Andria, Andriana,
Andriea, Andrieka,
Andrienne, Andrietta,
Andrina, Andris, Aundrea

Angel (Greek) a short form
of Angela.
Angell, Angil, Anjel

Angela (Greek) angel;
messenger.
Angala, Anganita, Ange,
Angel, Angelanell,
Angelanette, Angele,
Angèle, Angelea,
Angeleah, Angelee,
Angeleigh, Angeles,
Angeli, Angelia, Angelic,
Angelica, Angelina,
Angelique, Angelita,
Angella, Angelle,
Angellita, Angie, Anglea,
Anjela

Angelica (Greek) an alter-
nate form of Angela.
Angel, Angelici, Angelika,
Angeliki, Angellica,

Angilica, Anjelica,
Anjelika

Angelina, Angeline
(Russian) forms of Angela.
Angalena, Angalina,
Angeleen, Angelena,
Angelene, Angeliana,
Angeleana, Angellina,
Angelyn, Angelyna,
Angelyne, Angelynn,
Angelynne, Anhelina,
Anjelina

Angelique (French) a form
of Angela.
Angeliqua, Angélique,
Angilique, Anjelique

Angie (Greek) a familiar
form of Angela.
Angee, Angey, Angi, Angy

Anika (Czech) a familiar
form of Anna.
Anaka, Aneeky, Aneka,
Anekah, Anica, Anicka,
Anik, Anikah, Anikka,
Anikke, Aniko, Anneka,
Annik, Annika, Anouska,
Anuska

Anisha (English) a form
of Agnes, Ann.
Anis, Anisa, Anise, Anissa,
Annissa

Anita (Spanish) a form of
Ann, Anna. See also Nita.
Aneeta, Aneetah,
Aneethah, Anetha,
Anitha, Anithah, Anitia,
Anitra, Anitte

Ann, Anne (English)
gracious. A form of
Hannah.
An, Ana, Anelle, Anice,
Anikó, Anissa, Anita,
Anke, Annalie, Annchen,
Annette, Annie, Annik,
Annika, Annze, Anouche,
Anouk

Anna (German, Italian,
Czech, Swedish) gracious.
A form of Hannah.
Culture: Anna Pavlova
was a famous Russian
ballerina. See also Anika,
Anisha, Nina.
Ana, Anah, Ania, Anica,
Anita, Anja, Anka,
Annina, Annora, Anona,
Anya, Anyu, Aska

**Annemarie, Annmarie,
Anne-Marie** (English)
combinations of
Anne + Marie.
Annamaria, Anna-Maria,
Annamarie, Anna-Marie,
Annmaria

Annette (French) a form
of Ann.
Anet, Aneta, Anetra,
Anett, Anetta, Anette,
Anneth, Annett, Annetta

Annie (English) a familiar
form of Ann.
Anni, Anny

Annik, Annika (Russian)
forms of Ann.
Aneka, Anekah, Anica,
Anika, Anninka

Antoinette (French) a form
of Antonia. See also Toni.
Anta, Antanette,
Antoinella, Antoinet,
Antonella, Antonetta,
Antonette, Antonice,
Antonieta, Antonietta,
Antonique

Antonia (Greek) flourish-
ing. (Latin) praiseworthy.
A feminine form of
Anthony. See also Toni,
Tonya, Tosha.
Ansonia, Ansonya,
Antania, Antoinette,
Antona, Antoñía,
Antonice, Antonie,
Antonina, Antonine,
Antonnea, Antonnia,
Antonya

Anya (Russian) a form
of Anna.
Anja

April (Latin) opening.
Aprele, Aprelle, Apriell,
Aprielle, Aprila, Aprile,
Aprilette, Aprili, Aprill,
Apryl

Apryl (Latin) an alternate
form of April.
Apryle

Arabella (Latin) beautiful
altar.
Ara, Arabela, Arabele,
Arabelle, Belle

Aretha (Greek) virtuous.
Areatha, Areetha, Areta,
Aretina, Aretta, Arette,
Arita, Aritha, Retha, Ritha

Ariana, Arianna (Greek)
holy.
Aeriana, Aerianna,
Airiana, Arieana

Ariane (French), **Arianne**
(English) forms of Ariana,
Arianna.
Aeriann, Airiann, Ari,
Arianie, Ariann, Ariannie,
Arieann, Arien, Arienne,
Arieon, Aryane, Aryanna,
Aryanne

Ariel (Hebrew) lioness
of God.
Aeriale, Aeriel, Aeriela,
Aeryal, Aire, Aireal, Airial,
Ari, Aria, Arial, Ariale,
Arieal, Ariela, Arielle

Arielle (French) a form
of Ariel.
Aeriell, Ariella

Arin (Hebrew) enlightened.
(Arabic) messenger.
A feminine form of Aaron.
See also Erin.
Aaren, Arinn, Aryn

Arlene (Irish) pledge.
A feminine form of Arlen.
Arla, Arlana, Arleen,
Arleigh, Arlen, Arlena,
Arlenis, Arlette, Arleyne,
Arliene, Arlina, Arlinda,
Arline, Arlis, Arly, Arlyn,
Arlyne

Asha (Arabic, Swahili)
an alternate form of Aisha.
Ashia, Ashyah

Ashley (English) ash tree
meadow. See also Lee.
Ashala, Ashalee, Ashalei,
Ashaley, Ashelee, Ashelei,
Asheleigh, Asheley,
Ashely, Ashla, Ashlay,
Ashlea, Ashleah, Ashleay,
Ashlee, Ashlei, Ashleigh,
Ashli, Ashlie, Ashly, Ashlye

Ashlyn, Ashlynn (English)
ash tree pool. (Irish) vision,
dream.
Ashlan, Ashleann,
Ashleen, Ashleene,
Ashlen, Ashlene, Ashliann,
Ashlianne, Ashlin,
Ashline, Ashling, Ashlyne,
Ashlynne

Asia (Greek) resurrection.
(English) eastern sunrise.
(Swahili) an alternate form
of Aisha.
Aisia, Asiah, Asian, Asya,
Aysia, Aysiah, Aysian

Aspen (English) aspen tree.
Aspin, Aspyn

Athena (Greek) wise.
Mythology: the goddess
of wisdom.
Athenea, Athene, Athina,
Atina

Aubrey (German) noble;
bearlike. (French) blond
ruler; elf ruler.
Aubary, Auberi, Aubery,
Aubray, Aubre, Aubrea,
Aubreah, Aubree, Aubrei,
Aubreigh, Aubrette,

Aubria, Aubrie, Aubry,
Aubury

Aubrie (French) an alternate form of Aubrey.
Aubri

Audrey (English) noble strength.
Aude, Audey, Audi, Audie,
Audra, Audray, Audre,
Audree, Audreen, Audri,
Audria, Audrianna,
Audrianne, Audrie,
Audrin, Audrina, Audriya,
Audry, Audrye

Aurora (Latin) dawn.
Aurore, Ora, Ori, Orie,
Rora

Autumn (Latin) autumn.
Autum

Ava (Greek) an alternate form of Eva.
Avada, Avae, Ave, Aveen

Ayanna (Hindi) innocent.
Ayania

Ayesha (Persian) a form of Aisha.
Ayasha

Ayla (Hebrew) oak tree.
Aylana, Aylee, Ayleen,
Aylene, Aylie

B

Bailey (English) bailiff.
Bailee, Bailley, Baillie,
Bailly, Baily, Bali, Bayla,
Baylee, Baylie, Bayly

Bandi (Punjabi) prisoner.
Banda, Bandy

Barbara (Latin) stranger, foreigner.
Babara, Babb, Babbie,
Babe, Babette, Babina,
Babs, Barb, Barbara-Ann,
Barbarit, Barbarita,
Barbary, Barbeeleen,
Barbie, Barbora,
Barborka, Barbra,
Barbraann, Barbro, Bobbi,
Bobbie

Beatrice (Latin) blessed; happy; bringer of joy.
Bea, Beatrica, Béatrice,
Beatricia, Beatriks,
Beatris, Beatrisa, Beatrise,
Beatriss, Beatrissa,
Beatrix, Beatriz, Beattie,
Beatty, Bebe, Bee, Beitris,
Trice

Becky (American) a familiar form of Rebecca.
Becki, Beckie

Belinda (Spanish) beautiful. Literature: a name coined by English poet Alexander Pope in *The Rape of the Lock*. See also Linda.
Bel, Belindra, Belle, Belynda

Benita (Spanish) blessed.
Benetta, Benitta, Bennita, Neeta

Bernadette (French) brave as a bear. (English) a feminine form of Bernard.
Bera, Beradette, Berna, Bernadet, Bernadett, Bernadetta, Bernarda, Bernardette, Bernedet, Bernedette, Bernessa, Berneta

Bertha (German) bright; illustrious; brilliant ruler.
Barta, Bartha, Berlynn, Berta, Berte, Berthe, Bertita, Bertrona, Bertus

Beth (Hebrew, Aramaic) house of God. A short form of Bethany, Elizabeth.
Betha, Bethe, Bethia

Bethany (Aramaic) house of figs. Bible: a village near Jerusalem where Lazarus lived.
Beth, Bethane, Bethanee, Bethaney, Bethani, Bethania, Bethanie, Bethann, Bethanney, Bethannie, Bethanny, Bethena, Betheny, Bethia, Bethina, Bethney

Betsy (American) a familiar form of Elizabeth.
Betsey, Betsi, Betsie

Bettina (American) a combination of Beth + Tina.
Betina, Betine, Betti, Bettine

Betty (Hebrew) consecrated to God. (English) a familiar form of Elizabeth.
Bette, Bettye, Bettyjean, Betty-Jean, Bettyjo, Betty-Jo, Bettylou, Betty-Lou, Bety

Beverly (English) beaver field.
Bev, Bevalee, Bevan, Bevann, Bevanne, Bevany, Beverle, Beverlee, Beverley, Beverlie, Beverlyann, Bevlyn, Bevlynn, Bevlynne, Bevvy, Verly

Bianca (Italian) white. See also Blanca.
Bellanca, Beonca, Beyonca, Biancha, Biancia, Bianey, Binney, Bionca, Bioncha, Blanche

Billie (English) strong willed.
Bilee, Bili, Billi, Billy, Billye

Blair (Scottish) plains dweller.
Blaire, Blayre

Blanca (Italian) an alternate form of Bianca.
Bellanca, Blancka, Blanka

Blythe (English) happy, cheerful.
Blithe, Blyth

Bobbi, Bobbie (American) familiar forms of Barbara, Roberta.
Baubie, Bobbisue, Bobby, Bobbye, Bobi, Bobie

Bobbi-Jo (American) a combination of Bobbi + Jo.
Bobbiejo, Bobbie-Jo, Bobbijo, Bobby-Jo, Bobijo

Bonita (Spanish) pretty.
Bonnie, Bonny

Bonnie, Bonny (English, Scottish) beautiful, pretty. (Spanish) familiar forms of Bonita.
Boni, Bonie, Bonne, Bonnee, Bonnell, Bonnetta, Bonney, Bonni, Bonnin

Brandi, Brandie (Dutch) alternate forms of Brandy.
Brandice, Brandee, Brandii, Brandily, Brandin, Brandis, Brandise, Brani, Branndie

Brandy (Dutch) an after-dinner drink made from distilled wine.
Brand, Branda, Brandace, Brandaise, Brandala, Brande, Brandea,
Brandee, Brandei, Brandeli, Brandell, Brandi, Brandye, Brandylee, Brandy-Lee, Brandy-Leigh, Brandyn, Brann, Brantley, Branyell

Breana, Breanna (Irish) alternate forms of Briana.
Breanda, Bre-Anna, Breauna, Breawna, Breeana, Breeanna, Breeauna, Breiana, Breiann, Breila, Breina

Breann, Breanne (Irish) alternate forms of Briana.
Bre-Ann, Bre-Anne, Breaunne, Bree, Breean, Breeann, Breeanne, Breelyn, Breiann, Breighann, Brieann, Brieon

Bree (Irish) a short form of Breann. (English) broth. See also Brie.
Brea, Breah, Breay, Breea, Brei, Breigh

Brenda (Irish) little raven. (English) sword. A feminine form of Brendan.
Brendell, Brendelle, Brendette, Brendie, Brendyl

Brenna (Irish) an alternate form of Brenda.
Bren, Brenie, Brenin, Brenn, Brennah, Brennaugh

Brett (Irish) a short form of Britany.

Brett *(cont.)*
Bret, Bretta, Brette, Brettin, Bretton

Briana, Brianna (Irish)
strong; virtuous, honorable. Feminine forms
of Brian.
Brana, Breana, Breann, Bria, Briah, Briahna, Briand, Brianda, Briannah, Brianne, Brianni, Briannon, Briauna, Brina, Briona, Bryanna, Bryna

Brianne (Irish) an alternate
form of Briana.
Briane, Briann, Brienne, Bryanne, Bryn, Brynn, Brynne

Briar (French) heather.
Brear, Brier, Briet, Brieta, Brietta, Brya, Bryar

Bridget (Irish) strong.
Beret, Berget, Biddy, Birgitte, Bride, Bridey, Bridger, Bridgete, Bridgett, Bridgid, Bridgot, Brietta, Brigada, Briget, Brigid, Brigida, Brigitte, Brita

Bridgett, Bridgette (Irish)
alternate forms of Bridget.
Bridgitte, Brigette, Briggitte, Brigitta

Brie (French) a type
of cheese. Geography:
a region in France known
for its cheese. See also
Bree.

Brielle, Briena, Brieon, Briette

Brieanne (American)
a combination of Brie +
Ann.
Brieann, Brie-Ann, Brieanna, Brie-Anne

Brielle (French) a form
of Brie.

Brienne (French) a form
of Briana.
Brienn

Brigitte (French) a form
of Bridget.
Brigette, Briggitte, Brigit, Brigita

Britaney, Brittaney
(English) alternate forms
of Britany, Brittany.
Britanee, Britanny, Britenee, Briteny, Britianey, British, Britkney, Britley, Britlyn, Britney, Briton

Britani, Brittanie
(English) alternate forms
of Britany, Brittany.
Brit, Britania, Britanica, Britanie, Britanii, Britanni, Britannia, Britatani, Britia, Britini, Brittanni, Brittannia, Brittannie, Brittenie, Brittiani, Brittianni

Britany, Brittany (English)
from Britain. See also
Brett.

Brita, Britana, Britaney, Britani, Britanie, Britann, Britlyn, Britney, Britt, Brittainny, Brittainy, Brittamy, Brittan, Brittana, Brittane, Brittanee, Brittaney, Brittani, Brittania, Brittanica, Brittany-Ann, Brittanyne, Brittell, Britten, Brittenee, Britteney, Britteny, Brittiany, Brittlin, Brittlynn, Britton, Brittoni, Brittony, Bryttany

Britney, Brittney (English) alternate forms of Britany, Brittany.
Bittney, Bridnee, Bridney, Britnay, Britne, Britnee, Britnei, Britni, Britny, Britnye, Brittnay, Brittnaye, Brittne, Brittnea, Brittnee, Brittneigh, Brittny, Brytnea, Brytni

Britni, Brittni (English) alternate forms of Britney, Britney.
Britnie, Brittnie

Britt, Britta (Latin) short forms of Britany, Brittany. (Swedish) strong.
Brett, Brit, Brita, Britte

Bronwyn (Welsh) white breasted.
Bron, Bronia, Bronney, Bronnie, Bronny,

Bronwen, Bronwin, Bronwynn, Bronwynne, Bronya

Brooke (English) brook, stream.
Brook, Brookelle, Brookie, Brooks, Brooky

Bryanna, Bryanne (Irish) alternate forms of Briana.
Bryana, Bryann

Bryn, Brynn (Latin) from the boundary line. (Welsh) mound.
Brinn, Brynan, Brynee, Brynne

C

Cailin (American) a form of Caitlin.
Caileen, Cailene, Cailine, Cailyn, Cailynn, Cailynne, Cayleen, Caylene, Caylin, Cayline, Caylyn, Caylyne, Caylynne

Caitlin (Irish) pure. An alternate form of Cathleen. See also Kaitlin, Katelin.
Caeley, Cailey, Cailin, Caitlan, Caitland, Caitlandt, Caitleen, Caitlen, Caitlene, Caitline, Caitlinn, Caitlon, Caitlyn, Caitria, Caitriona, Catlee,

Caitlin *(cont.)*
Catleen, Catleene, Catlin, Cayley

Caitlyn (Irish) an alternate form of Caitlin. See also Kaitlyn.
Caitlynn, Caitlynne, Catlyn, Catlynn, Catlynne

Calandra (Greek) lark.
Caelan, Cailan, Calan, Calandria, Caleida, Calendra, Calendre, Caylan, Kalan, Kalandra, Kalandria

Caleigh, Caley (American) alternate forms of Kayley, Kaylie, Kelly.

Cali, Calli (Greek) alternate forms of Callie. See also Kali.

Callie (Greek, Arabic) beautiful. See also Cayla, Kalli.
Cal, Caleigh, Caley, Cali, Calie, Callee, Calley, Calli, Cally

Calvina (Latin) bald. A feminine form of Calvin.
Calvine, Calvinetta, Calvinette

Cameron (Scottish) crooked nose.
Camera, Cameran, Cameren, Cameri, Cameria, Camesha, Cameshia, Cami

Cami, Cammie (French) short forms of Camille. See also Kami.
Camey, Camie, Cammi, Cammy, Cammye

Camilla (Italian) a form of Camille.
Camia, Camila, Camillia, Chamelea, Chamelia, Chamika, Chamila, Chamilia

Camille (French) young ceremonial attendant.
Cam, Cami, Camill, Camilla, Cammille, Cammillie, Cammilyn, Cammyl, Cammyll, Camylle, Chamelle, Chamille, Kamille

Candace (Greek) glittering white; glowing. History: the name and title of the queens of ancient Ethiopia. See also Kandace.
Cace, Canace, Canda, Candas, Candelle, Candi, Candice, Candida, Candis, Candyce

Candi, Candy (American) familiar forms of Candace, Candice.
Candee, Candie

Candice, Candis, Candyce (Greek) alternate forms of Candace.
Candes, Candi, Candias, Candies, Candise, Candiss, Candus, Candys, Candyse, Cyndyss

Candra (Latin) glowing.
Candrea, Candria, Kandra

Caprice (Italian) fanciful.
Cappi, Caprece, Capricia, Caprina, Caprise, Capritta

Cara (Latin) dear. (Irish) friend. See also Karah.
Caragh, Carah, Caralea, Caralee, Caralia, Caralie, Caralin, Caraline, Caralyn, Caranda, Carey, Carra

Carey (Welsh) a familiar form of Cara, Caroline, Karen, Katherine. See also Carrie, Kari.
Caree, Cari, Carrey, Cary

Cari, Carie (Welsh) alternate forms of Carey, Kari.

Carina (Greek) a familiar form of Cora. (Italian) dear little one. (Swedish) a form of Karen.
Carena, Carin, Carine, Caryn

Carissa (Greek) beloved.
Caressa, Carisa, Carrissa, Charisa, Charissa, Karissa

Carla (Latin) an alternate form of Carol, Caroline. (German) farmer. (English) strong and womanly.
Carila, Carilla, Carlan, Carle, Carleah, Carleigh, Carlene, Carleta, Carletha, Carlethe, Carlia, Carlicia, Carliqua, Carlissa, Carlita, Carliyle, Carlonda, Carlotta, Carlreca, Carlye,

Carlyjo, Carlyle, Carlyse, Carlysle

Carlee, Carley (English) alternate forms of Carly.

Carlene (English) a form of Caroline.
Carlaen, Carlaena, Carleen, Carleena, Carlen, Carlena, Carlenna, Carline, Carlyne, Karlene

Carli, Carlie (English) alternate forms of Carly. See also Karli.

Carlin, Carlyn (Latin) short forms of Caroline. (Irish) little champion.
Carlen, Carlina, Carlinda, Carline, Carrlin, Carlyne

Carly (English) a familiar form of Caroline, Charlotte. See also Karli.
Carlee, Carley, Carli, Carlie, Carlye

Carmela, Carmella (Hebrew) garden; vineyard. Bible: Mount Carmel in Israel is often thought of as paradise.
Carma, Carmaletta, Carmalit, Carmalita, Carmalla, Carmarit, Carmel, Carmeli, Carmelia, Carmelina, Carmelit, Carmelita, Carmelitha, Carmelitia, Carmelle, Carmellia, Carmellina, Carmellit, Carmellita, Carmellitha, Carmellitia, Carmesa,

Carmela, Carmella *(cont.)*
Carmesha, Carmi, Carmie,
Carmiel, Carmil, Carmila,
Carmilla, Carmisha,
Leeta, Lita

Carmen (Latin) song.
Religion: Santa Maria
del Carmen—Saint Mary
of Mount Carmel—is one
of the titles of the Virgin
Mary. See also Karmen.
Carma, Carmaine,
Carman, Carmelina,
Carmelita, Carmencita,
Carmene, Carmi, Carmia,
Carmin, Carmina,
Carmine, Carmita,
Carmon, Carmynn,
Charmaine

Carol (German) farmer.
(French) song of joy.
(English) strong and
womanly. A feminine
form of Carl, Charles.
See also Carlene,
Charlene, Charlotte.
Carel, Carely, Cariel,
Carilis, Carilise, Carilyse,
Carle, Carley, Carlita,
Caro, Carola, Carole,
Caroleen, Carolenia,
Carolinda, Caroline,
Caroll, Carolyn, Carrie,
Carrol, Carroll, Caryl

Carole (English) an alternate form of Carol.
Carolee, Karole, Karrole

Carolina (Italian) a form
of Caroline.
Carilena, Carlena,
Carlina, Carlita, Carlota,
Carrolena, Karolina

Caroline (French) little and
womanly. See also Carla.
Caralin, Caraline,
Carileen, Carilene, Carilin,
Cariline, Carling, Carly,
Caro, Carolann, Carolin,
Carolina, Carrie,
Carroleen, Carrolene,
Carrolin, Carroline, Cary,
Charlene

Carolyn (English) a form of
Caroline. See also Karolyn.
Caralyn, Caralynn,
Caralynne, Carilyn,
Carilynn, Carilynne,
Carlyn, Carlynn, Carlynne,
Carolyne, Carolynn,
Carolynne, Carrolyn,
Carrolynn, Carrolynne

Carra (Irish) an alternate
form of Cara.

Carrie (English) a familiar
form of Carol, Caroline.
See also Carey, Kari, Karri.
Carree, Carri, Carria,
Carry

Caryn (Danish) a form
of Karen.
Caren, Caron, Caronne,
Carren, Carrin, Carron,
Caryna, Caryne, Carynn

Casey (Irish) brave.
See also Kasey.
Cacy, Cascy, Casie, Cass,
Casse, Cassee, Cassey,

Cassye, Casy, Cayce,
Cayse, Caysee, Caysy

Casie (Irish) an alternate
form of Casey.
Caci, Casci, Cascie, Casi,
Cass, Cayci, Caysi, Caysie,
Cazzi

Cassandra (Greek) helper
of men. Mythology:
a prophetess of ancient
Greece whose prophesies
were not believed. See
also Kassandra, Sandra,
Sandy.
Casandra, Casandre,
Casandrey, Casandri,
Casandria, Casaundra,
Casaundria, Casondra,
Casondre, Casondria,
Cass, Cassandre,
Cassandri, Cassandry,
Cassaundra, Cassaundre,
Cassaundri, Cassie,
Cassondra, Cassondre,
Cassondri, Cassondria,
Cassundra, Cassundre

Cassidy (Irish) clever.
See also Kassidy.
Casadee, Casadi, Casadie,
Cass, Cassadi, Cassadie,
Cassadina, Cassady,
Casseday, Cassiddy,
Cassidee, Cassidi, Cassidie,
Cassity

Cassie (Greek) a familiar
form of Cassandra,
Catherine. See also Kassie.
Cassey, Cassi, Cassy

Catalina (Spanish) a form
of Catherine.
Cataleen, Catalena,
Catalene, Catalin,
Catalyn, Catalyna,
Cateline, Kataleena,
Katalina, Katalyn

Catherine (Greek) pure.
(English) a form of
Katherine.
Cat, Catalina, Catarina,
Catarine, Cate, Caterina,
Catha, Cathann,
Cathanne, Catharina,
Catharine, Cathenne,
Catheren, Catherene,
Catheria, Catherin,
Catherina, Catheryn,
Cathi, Cathleen, Cathrine,
Cathryn, Cathy, Catlaina,
Catreeka, Catrelle,
Catrice, Catricia, Catrika,
Catrin, Catrina, Catryn,
Catteeka, Cattiah

Cathi, Cathy (Greek)
familiar forms of
Catherine, Cathleen.
See also Kathi, Kathy.
Catha, Cathe, Cathee,
Cathey, Cathie

Cathleen (Irish) a form
of Catherine. See also
Caitlin, Katelin, Kathleen.
Cathaleen, Cathelin,
Cathelina, Cathelyn,
Cathi, Cathleana,
Cathlene, Cathleyn,
Cathlin, Cathlyn,
Cathlyne, Cathy

Cathrine, Cathryn
(Greek) alternate forms
of Catherine.

Catrina (Slavic) a form
of Catherine, Katrina.
**Catina, Catreen, Catreena,
Catrene, Catrenia,
Catrine, Catrinia,
Catriona, Catroina**

Cayla (Hebrew) an alter-
nate form of Kayla.
**Cailee, Cailey, Cailie, Caily,
Calee, Caly, Caylee, Cayley,
Caylie, Cayly**

Cecilia (Latin) blind.
A feminine form of Cecil.
See also Sheila.
**Cacelia, Cacilia, Cacilie,
Caecilia, Cece, Ceceilia,
Ceceli, Cecelia, Cecely,
Cecelyn, Cecette, Cecil,
Cecila, Cecile, Cecilea,
Ceciley, Cecilija, Cecilla,
Cecille, Cecillia, Cecily,
Ceclia, Cecylia, Cee, Ceil,
Ceila, Ceilagh, Ceileh,
Ceileigh, Ceilena, Celia,
Cescelia, Cescelie, Cescily,
Cesia, Cesya, Cicelia,
Cicely, Cilley, Secilia, Selia**

Celena (Greek) an alternate
form of Selena.
**Celeen, Celeena, Celene,
Celenia**

Celeste (Latin) celestial,
heavenly.
**Cele, Celense, Celes,
Celesia, Celesley, Celest,
Celesta, Celestia,**

**Celestial, Celestin,
Celestina, Celestine,
Celestinia, Celestyn,
Celestyna, Celina, Celine,
Selestina**

Celia (Latin) a short form
of Cecilia.
Ceilia, Celle

Celina (Greek) an alternate
form of Celena.
**Caleena, Calena, Calina,
Celena, Celinda, Celinka,
Celka, Selina**

Celine (Greek) an alternate
form of Celena.
**Caline, Celeen, Celene,
Céline, Cellina, Cellinn**

Chanda (Sanskrit) great
goddess. Religion: the
name assumed by the
Hindu goddess Devi.
See also Shanda.
**Chandee, Chandey,
Chandi, Chandie**

Chandra (Sanskrit) moon.
Religion: one of the names
of the Hindu goddess
Shakti. See also Shandra.
**Chandre, Chandrea,
Chandrelle, Chandria**

Chanel (English) channel.
See also Shanel.
**Chaneel, Chaneil, Chanell,
Chanelle, Channel**

Chanell, Chanelle
(English) alternate forms
of Chanel.
Shanell

Chantal (French) song.
See also Shanta.
Chandal, Chanta,
Chantaal, Chantae,
Chantael, Chantai,
Chantale, Chantall,
Chantalle, Chantara,
Chantarai, Chantasia,
Chantay, Chantaye,
Chanteau, Chantel,
Chantiel, Chantielle,
Chantil, Chantila,
Chantill, Chantille,
Chantle, Chantoya,
Chantra, Chantri,
Chantrice, Chantrill,
Chaunta, Chauntay

Chantel, Chantelle
(French) alternate forms
of Chantal. See also
Shantel.
Chante, Chantea,
Chantee, Chantée,
Chanteese, Chantela,
Chantele, Chantell,
Chantella, Chanter,
Chantey, Chantez,
Chantrel, Chantrell,
Chantrelle, Chantress,
Chaunte, Chauntea,
Chauntéa, Chauntee,
Chauntel, Chauntell,
Chauntelle, Chawntel,
Chawntell, Chawntelle,
Chontelle

Chardae, Charde
(Punjabi) charitable.
See also Shardae.

Charda, Chardai, Charday,
Chardea, Chardee,
Chardée, Chardese

Charis (Greek) grace;
kindness.
Chari, Charice, Charle,
Charish, Charisse

Charissa, Charisse
(Greek) forms of Charity.
Charesa, Charese, Charis,
Charisa, Charise,
Charisha, Charissee,
Charista

Charity (Latin) charity,
kindness.
Carisa, Carisia, Carissa,
Carita, Chariety, Charis,
Charissa, Charisse,
Charista, Charita, Chariti,
Sharity

Charla (French, English)
a short form of Charlene,
Charlotte.
Char

Charlene (English) little
and womanly. A form
of Caroline. See also
Carol, Karla, Sharlene.
Charla, Charlaina,
Charlaine, Charleen,
Charleesa, Charlena,
Charlesena, Charline,
Charlyn, Charlyne,
Charlynn, Charlynne,
Charlzina

Charlie (German, English)
strong and womanly. A
feminine form of Charles.

Charlie (cont.)
Charla, Charle, Charlea, Charlee, Charleigh, Charley, Charli, Charyl, Chatty, Sharli, Sharlie

Charlotte (French) little and womanly. A form of Caroline. Literature: Charlotte Brontë was a British novelist and poet best known for her novel *Jane Eyre*.
Carla, Carlotta, Carly, Char, Chara, Charil, Charl, Charla, Charle, Charlene, Charlet, Charlett, Charletta, Charlette, Charlie, Charlisa, Charlita, Charlott, Charlotta, Charlotty, Charmaine, Charo, Charolet, Charolette, Charoline, Charolot, Charolotte

Charmaine (French) a form of Carmen.
Charamy, Charma, Charmain, Charmalique, Charman, Charmane, Charmar, Charmara, Charmayane, Charmeen, Charmene, Charmese, Charmian, Charmin, Charmine, Charmion, Charmisa, Charmon, Charmyn

Chasity, Chassidy (Latin) alternate forms of Chastity.
Chasa Dee, Chasadie, Chasady, Chasidy, Chasiti, **Chassedi, Chassey, Chassie, Chassity, Chassy**

Chastity (Latin) pure.
Chasity, Chasta, Chastady, Chastidy, Chastin, Chastitie, Chastney, Chasty

Chelsea (English) seaport. See also Kelsi.
Chelese, Chelesia, Chelsa, Chelsae, Chelse, Chelsee, Chelsei, Chelsey, Chelsie, Chesea, Cheslee

Chelsey (English) an alternate form of Chelsea. See also Kelsey.
Chelcy, Chelsay, Chelsy, Chesley

Chelsie (English) an alternate form of Chelsea.
Chelcie, Chelli, Chellie, Chellise, Chellsie, Chelsi, Chelsia, Cheslie, Chessie

Cherelle, Cherrelle (French) alternate forms of Cheryl. See also Sherell.
Charell, Charelle

Cheri, Cherie (French) familiar forms of Cheryl.
Cher, Chérie

Cherise (French) a form of Cherish.
Charisa, Charise, Cherece, Chereese, Cheresa, Cherese, Cheresse, Cherice

Cherish (English) dearly held, precious.
Charish, Charisha, Cheerish, Cherise,

Cherishe, Cherrish, Sherish

Cheryl (French) beloved. See also Sheryl.
Charel, Charil, Charyl, Cherelle, Cherilyn, Cherrelle, Cheryl-Ann, Cheryl-Anne, Cheryle, Cherylee, Cherylene, Cheryll, Cherylle, Cheryl-Lee, Cheryline, Cheryn

Cheyenne (Cheyenne) a tribal name.
Chey, Cheyan, Cheyana, Cheyann, Cheyanne, Cheyene, Cheyenna, Chi, Chi-Anna, Chie, Chyann, Chyanna, Chyanne

Chiquita (Spanish) little one.
Chaqueta, Chaquita, Chica, Chickie, Chicky, Chikata, Chikita, Chiqueta, Chiquila, Chiquite, Chiquitha, Chiquithe, Chiquitia, Chiquitta

Chloe (Greek) blooming, verdant. Mythology: the goddess of agriculture.
Chloé, Chlöe, Chloee, Clo, Cloe, Cloey, Kloe

Chrissy (English) a familiar form of Christina.
Chrisie, Chrissee, Chrissie, Crissie, Khrissy

Christa (German) a short form of Christina. History: Christa McAuliffe, an American school teacher, was the first civilian on a U.S. space flight. See also Krista.
Chrysta, Crista, Crysta

Christal (Latin) an alternate form of Crystal. (Scottish) a form of Christina.
Christalene, Christalin, Christaline, Christall, Christalle, Christalyn, Christel, Christelle, Chrystal

Christen, Christin (Greek) alternate forms of Christina.
Christan, Christyn, Chrystan, Chrysten, Chrystin, Chrystyn, Crestienne, Kristen

Christi, Christie (Greek) short forms of Christina, Christine.
Christy, Chrysti, Chrystie, Chrysty, Kristi

Christian, Christiana (Greek) alternate forms of Christina. See also Kristian.
Christiane, Christiann, Christi-Ann, Christianna, Christianne, Christi-Anne, Christianni, Christienne, Christy-Ann, Christy-Anne, Chrystyann, Chrystyanne, Crystiann, Crystianne

Christin (Greek) a short form of Christina.
Christen

Christina (Greek) Christian; anointed. See also Kristina, Tina.
Chris, Chrissa, Chrissy, Christa, Christeena, Christella, Christena, Christi, Christian, Christiana, Christie, Christin, Christine, Christinea, Christinna, Christna, Christy, Christyna, Chrys, Chrystena, Chrystina, Chrystyna, Cristeena, Cristena, Cristina, Cristy, Crystal, Crystina, Crystyna

Christine (French, English) forms of Christina. See also Kirsten, Kristen, Kristine.
Chrisa, Christeen, Christen, Christene, Christi, Christie, Christin, Christy, Chrys, Chrystine, Cristeen, Cristene, Cristine, Crystine

Christy (English) a short form of Christina, Christine.
Cristy

Ciara, Cierra (Irish) black. See also Sierra.
Ceara, Cearaa, Cearia, Cearra, Cera, Ciaara, Ciarra, Ciarrah, Cieara, Ciearra, Ciearria, Ciera, Cierrah

Cindy (Greek) moon. (Latin) a familiar form of Cynthia.
Cindee, Cindi, Cindl, Cynda, Cyndal, Cyndale, Cyndall, Cyndee, Cyndel, Cyndi, Cyndia, Cyndie, Cyndle, Cyndy

Claire (French) a form of Clara.
Clair, Clairette, Klaire, Klarye

Clara (Latin) clear; bright. Music: Clara Shumann was a famous nineteenth-century German composer.
Claire, Clarabelle, Clare, Claresta, Clarette, Clarey, Clari, Claribel, Clarice, Clarie, Clarina, Clarinda, Clarine, Clarissa, Clarita, Claritza, Clarizza, Clary

Clare (English) a form of Clara.

Clarissa (Greek) brilliant. (Italian) a form of Clara.
Clarecia, Claresa, Claressa, Claresta, Clarisa, Clarissia, Clarrisa, Clarrissa, Clerissa

Claudia (Latin) lame. A feminine form of Claude. See also Gladys.
Claudee, Claudeen, Claudelle, Claudette, Claudex, Claudiane, Claudie, Claudie-Anne, Claudina, Claudine

Codi, Cody (English)
cushion.
**Coady, Codee, Codey,
Codie, Kodi**

Colby (English) coal town.
Geography: a region in
England known for
cheese-making.
**Cobi, Cobie, Colbi, Colbie,
Kolby**

Coleen, Colleen (Irish) girl.
**Coe, Coel, Cole, Colena,
Colene, Coley, Colina,
Colinda, Coline, Colleene,
Collen, Collene, Collie,
Collina, Colline, Colly**

Colette (Greek, French)
a familiar form of Nicole.
**Coe, Coetta, Coletta,
Collet, Collete, Collett,
Colletta, Collette, Kolette,
Kollette**

Connie (Latin) a familiar
form of Constance.
**Con, Connee, Conni,
Conny, Konnie, Konny**

Constance (Latin)
constant; firm. History:
Constance Motley was
the first African American
woman to be appointed
as a U.S. federal judge.
**Connie, Constancia,
Constancy, Constanta,
Constantia, Constantina,
Constantine, Constanza,
Konstance**

Cora (Greek) maiden.
Mythology: the daughter
of Demeter, the goddess
of agriculture.
**Coralee, Coretta, Corey,
Corissa, Corey, Corra, Kora**

Coral (Latin) coral.
**Corabel, Corabella,
Corabelle, Coralee,
Coraline, Coralyn, Corral,
Koral**

Corey, Cory (Greek) famil-
iar forms of Cora. (Irish)
from the hollow. See also
Kori.
**Coree, Cori, Correy,
Correye, Corry**

Cori, Corie, Corrie (Irish)
alternate forms of Corey.
**Corian, Coriann, Cori-Ann,
Corianne, Corri, Corrie-
Ann, Corrie-Anne**

Corina, Corinna (Greek)
familiar forms of Corinne.
**Coreena, Corinda,
Correna, Corrina,
Corrinna, Korina**

Corinne (Greek) maiden
**Coreen, Coren, Corin,
Corina, Corinda, Corine,
Corinee, Corinn, Corinna,
Correen, Corren,
Corrianne, Corrin,
Corrinn, Corrinne, Corryn,
Coryn, Corynn, Corynna**

Corissa (Greek) a familiar
form of Cora.
**Coresa, Coressa, Corisa,
Korissa**

Cortney (English) an alternate form of Courtney.
Cortnea, Cortnee, Cortneia, Cortni, Cortnie, Cortny, Corttney

Courtenay (English) an alternate form of Courtney.
Courteney

Courtney (English) from the court. See also Kortney, Kourtney.
Cortney, Courtena, Courtenay, Courtene, Courtnae, Courtnay, Courtnee, Courtnée, Courtnei, Courtni, Courtnie, Courtny, Courtonie

Crista (Italian) a form of Christa.

Cristen, Cristin (Irish) forms of Christen, Christin. See also Kristin.
Cristan, Cristyn, Crystan, Crysten, Crystin, Crystyn

Cristina (Greek) an alternate form of Christina. See also Kristina.
Cristiona, Cristy

Cristy (English) a familiar form of Cristina. An alternate form of Christy. See also Kristy.
Cristey, Cristi, Cristie, Crysti, Crystie, Crysty

Crystal (Latin) clear, brilliant glass. See also Krystal.
Christal, Chrystal, Chrystal-Lynn, Chrystel, Cristal, Cristalie, Cristalina, Cristalle, Cristel, Cristela, Cristelia, Cristella, Cristelle, Cristhie, Cristle, Crystala, Crystal-Ann, Crystal-Anne, Crystale, Crystalee, Crystalin, Crystall, Crystaly, Crystel, Crystelia, Crysthelle, Crystl, Crystle, Crystol, Crystole, Crystyl

Cynthia (Greek) moon. Mythology: another name for Artemis, the moon goddess.
Cindy, Cyneria, Cynethia, Cynithia, Cynthea, Cynthiana, Cynthiann, Cynthie, Cynthria, Cynthy, Cynthya, Cyntreia, Cythia

D

Daisy (English) day's eye. Botany: a white and yellow flower.
Dacey, Daisee, Daisey, Daisi, Daisia, Daisie, Dasey, Dasi, Dasie, Dasy, Daysee, Daysie, Daysy

Dakota (Native American) tribal name.

**Dakotah, Dakotha,
Dekoda, Dekota, Dekotah,
Dekotha**

Dale (English) valley.
**Dael, Dahl, Daile,
Daleleana, Dalena,
Dalina, Dayle**

Dallas (Irish) wise.
**Dalishya, Dalisia, Dalissia,
Dallys, Dalyce, Dalys**

Damaris (Greek) gentle
girl.
**Damar, Damara,
Damarius, Damary,
Damarys, Dameress,
Dameris, Damiris,
Dammaris, Dammeris,
Damris, Demaras, Demaris**

Dana (English) from
Denmark; bright as day.
**Daina, Dainna, Danae,
Danah, Danai, Danaia,
Danalee, Danan, Danarra,
Danayla, Dane, Danean,
Danee, Daniah, Danie,
Danja, Danna, Dayna**

Danae (Greek) Mythology:
the mother of Perseus.
**Danaë, Danay, Danayla,
Danays, Danea, Danee,
Dannae, Denae, Denee**

Danelle (Hebrew) an alter-
nate form of Danielle.
**Danael, Danalle, Danel,
Danele, Danell, Danella,
Donelle, Donnelle**

Danette (American) a form
of Danielle.
Danetra, Danett, Danetta

Dani (Hebrew) a familiar
form of Danielle.
**Danee, Danie, Danne,
Dannee, Danni, Dannie,
Danny, Dannye, Dany**

Dania, Danya (Hebrew)
short forms of Danielle.
Daniah

Danica, Danika (Hebrew)
alternate forms of Danielle.
(Slavic) morning star.
**Daneeka, Danikla,
Danneeka, Dannica,
Dannika**

Daniella (Italian) a form
of Danielle.
Daniela, Dannilla, Danijela

Danielle (Hebrew, French)
God is my judge. A femi-
nine form of Daniel.
**Danae, Daneen, Daneil,
Daneille, Danelle, Dani,
Danial, Danialle, Danica,
Danie, Danielan, Daniele,
Danielka, Daniell,
Daniella, Danilka, Danille,
Danit, Danniele, Danniell,
Danniella, Dannielle,
Danya, Danyel, Donniella**

Danna (Hebrew) a short
form of Daniella. (English)
an alternate form of Dana.
**Danka, Dannae, Dannah,
Danne, Danni, Dannia,
Dannon, Danya**

Danyel, Danyell
(American) forms
of Danielle.
**Daniyel, Danya, Danyae,
Danyail, Danyaile, Danyal,
Danyale, Danyea, Danyele,
Danyella, Danyelle,
Danyle, Donnyale,
Donnyell, Donyale,
Donyell**

Daphne (Greek) laurel tree.
**Dafny, Daphane,
Daphaney, Daphanie,
Daphany, Dapheney,
Daphna, Daphnee,
Daphney, Daphnie,
Daphnique, Daphnit,
Daphny**

Dara (Hebrew)
compassionate.
**Dahra, Darah, Daraka,
Daralea, Daralee, Darda,
Darice, Darilyn, Darilyn,
Darisa, Darissa, Darja,
Darra, Darrah**

Darby (Irish) free.
(Scandinavian) deer estate.
**Darb, Darbi, Darbie,
Darbra**

Darci, Darcy (Irish) dark.
(French) fortress.
**Darcee, Darcelle, Darcey,
Darcie, Darsey, Darsi,
Darsie**

Daria (Greek) wealthy.
A feminine form of Darius.
**Dari, Darian, Darianne,
Darria, Darya**

Darla (English) a short
form of Darlene.
**Darli, Darlice, Darlie,
Darlis, Darly, Darlys**

Darlene (French) little dar-
ling. See also Daryl.
**Darilynn, Darla, Darlean,
Darleen, Darlena,
Darlenia, Darletha, Darlin,
Darline, Darling**

Daryl (French) a short form
of Darlene. (English)
beloved.
**Darelle, Darielle, Daril,
Darilynn, Darrel, Darrell,
Darrelle, Darreshia,
Darryl, Darryll**

Davina (Hebrew) beloved.
**Dava, Davannah, Davean,
Davee, Daveen, Daveena,
Davene, Daveon, Davey,
Davi, Daviana, Davie,
Davin, Davine, Davineen,
Davinia, Davinna,
Davonna, Davria, Devean,
Deveen, Devene, Devina**

Dawn (English) sunrise,
dawn.
**Dawana, Dawandrea,
Dawanna, Dawin, Dawna,
Dawne, Dawnee,
Dawnele, Dawnell,
Dawnelle, Dawnetta,
Dawnisha, Dawnlynn,
Dawnn, Dawnrae,
Dawnyel, Dawnyella,
Dawnyelle**

Dawna (English) an alternate form of Dawn.
Dawnna, Dawnya

Dayna (Scandinavian) a form of Dana.
Dayne, Daynna

Deana (Latin) divine. (English) valley. A feminine form of Dean.
Deane, Deanielle, Deanisha, Deanna, Deena

Deandra (American) a combination of Dee + Andrea.
Deandre, Deandré, Deandrea, Deandree, Deandria, Deanndra, Diandra, Diandre, Diandrea

Deanna (Latin) an alternate form of Deana, Diana.
De, Dea, Deaana, Deahana, Deandra, Deandre, Deann, Déanna, Deannia, Deeanna, Deena

Deanne (Latin) an alternate form of Diane.
Dea, Deahanne, Deane, Deann, Déanne, Dee, Deeann, Deeanne

Debbie (Hebrew) a short form of Deborah.
Debbee, Debbey, Debbi, Debby, Debee, Debi, Debie

Deborah (Hebrew) bee. Bible: a great Hebrew prophetess.
Deb, Debbie, Debbora, Debborah, Deberah, Debor, Debora, Deboran, Deborha, Deborrah, Debra, Debrea, Debrena, Debria, Debrina, Debroah, Devora, Dobra

Debra (American) a short form of Deborah.
Debbra, Debbrah, Debrah

Dedra (American) a form of Deirdre.
Deeddra, Deedra, Deedrea, Deedrie

Deena (American) a form of Deana, Dena.

Deidra, Deidre (Irish) alternate forms of Deirdre.
Dedra, Deidrea, Deidrie, Diedra, Diedre, Dierdra

Deirdre (Irish) sorrowful; wanderer.
Dedra, Dee, Deerdra, Deerdre, Deidra, Deidre, Deirdree, Didi, Dierdre, Diérdre, Dierdrie

Delia (Greek) visible; from Delos. (German, Welsh) a short form of Adelaide. Mythology: a festival of Apollo held every five years in ancient Greece.
Dee, Dehlia, Del, Delea, Deli, Delinda, Dellia, Dellya, Delya

Delilah (Hebrew) brooder. Bible: the companion of Samson. See also Lila.

Delilah *(cont.)*
Dalia, Dalialah, Dalila, Daliliah, Delila, Delilia

Della a short form of Adelaide.
Del, Dela, Dell, Delle, Delli, Dellie, Dells

Delores (Spanish) an alternate form of Dolores.
Del, Delora, Delore, Deloria, Delories, Deloris, Delorise, Delorita

Demetria (Greek) cover of the earth. Mythology: Demeter was the Greek goddess of the harvest.
Deitra, Demeta, Demeteria, Demetra, Demetrice, Demetris, Demi, Demita, Demitra, Dymitra

Demi (Greek) a short form of Demetria. (French) half.
Demiah

Dena (Hebrew) an alternate form of Dina. (English, Native American) valley. See also Deana.
Deane, Deena, Deeyn, Denae, Dene, Denea, Deney, Denna

Denae (Hebrew) an alternate form of Dena.
Denaé, Denay, Denee, Deneé

Denise (French) Mythology: follower of Dionysus, the god of wine. A feminine form of Dennis.
Danice, Danise, Denese, Deney, Deni, Denica, Denice, Denie, Deniece, Denisha, Denisse, Denize, Denni, Dennie, Dennise, Denny, Dennys, Denyce, Denys, Denyse, Dinnie, Dinny

Denisha (American) a form of Denise.
Deneesha, Deneichia, Denesha, Deneshia, Deniesha, Denishia

Desiree (French) desired, longed for.
Desara, Desarae, Desarai, Desaraie, Desaray, Desare, Desaré, Desarea, Desaree, Desarie, Desera, Deserae, Deserai, Deseray, Desere, Deseree, Deseret, Deseri, Deserie, Deserrae, Deserray, Deserré, Desi, Desirae, Desirah, Desirai, Desiray, Desire, Desirea, Desirée, Désirée, Desirey, Desiri, Desray, Desree, Dessie, Dessirae, Dessire, Dezarae, Dezeray, Dezere, Dezerea, Dezerie, Dezirae, Deziree, Dezirée, Dezorae, Dezra, Dezrae, Dezyrae

Destiny (French) fate.
Desnine, Desta, Destanee, Destanie, Destannie, Destany, Desteni, Destin,

Destinee, Destinée, Destiney, Destini, Destinie, Destnie, Desty, Destyn, Destyne, Destyni

Devin (Irish) poet. An alternate form of Devon.
Devan, Devane, Devanie, Devany, Deven, Devena, Devenje, Deveny, Deveyn, Devina, Devine, Devinne, Devyn

Devon (English) from Devonshire.
Devonne

Diamond (Latin) precious gem.
Diamonda, Diamonia, Diamonique, Diamonte, Diamontina

Diana (Latin) divine. Mythology: the goddess of the hunt, the moon, and fertility. See also Deanna, Deanne.
Daiana, Daianna, Dayana, Dayanna, Di, Dia, Dianah, Dianalyn, Dianarose, Dianatris, Dianca, Diandra, Diane, Dianelis, Diania, Dianielle, Dianita, Dianna, Dianys, Didi, Dina

Diane (Latin) an alternate form of Diana.
Deane, Deanne, Deeane, Deeanne, Di, Dia, Diahann, Dian, Diani, Dianie, Diann, Dianne

Dianna (Latin) an alternate form of Diana.
Diahanna

Dina (Hebrew) vindicated.
Dinah

Dionne (Greek) divine queen. Mythology: the mother of Aphrodite, the goddess of love.
Deona, Deondra, Deonia, Deonjala, Deonna, Deonne, Deonyia, Dion, Diona, Diondra, Diondrea, Dione, Dionee, Dionis, Dionna, Dionte

Dixie (French) tenth. (English) wall; dike. Geography: a nickname for the American South.
Dix, Dixee, Dixi, Dixy

Dolores (Spanish) sorrowful. Religion: Santa Maria de los Dolores—Saint Mary of the Sorrows—is a name for the Virgin Mary. See also Lola.
Delores, Deloria, Dolly, Dolorcitas, Dolorita, Doloritas

Dominique, Domonique (French) belonging to the Lord.
Domanique, Domeneque, Domenique, Domineque, Dominiqua, Domino, Dominoque, Dominuque, Domique, Domminique, Domoniqua

Donna (Italian) lady.
Doña, Dondi, Donnaica,
Donnalee, Donnalen,
Donnay, Donnell,
Donnella, Donni, Donnica,
Donnie, Donnika,
Donnise, Donnisha,
Donnita, Donny, Dontia,
Donya

Dora (Greek) gift.
Doralia, Doralie, Doralisa,
Doraly, Doralynn, Doran,
Dorchen, Dore, Dorece,
Doree, Doreece, Doreen,
Dorelia, Dorella, Dorelle,
Doresha, Doressa,
Doretta, Dori, Dorika,
Doriley, Dorilis, Dorinda,
Dorion, Dorita, Doro,
Dory

Doreen (Greek) an
alternate form of Dora.
(Irish) moody, sullen.
(French) golden.
Doreena, Dorena, Dorene,
Dorina, Dorine

Doris (Greek) sea.
Mythology: the wife of
Nereus and mother of the
Nereids, or sea nymphs.
Dori, Dorice, Dorisa,
Dorise, Dorris, Dorrise,
Dorrys, Dory, Dorys

Dorothy (Greek) gift
of God. See also Thea.
Dasha, Dasya, Do, Doa,
Doe, Dolly, Dorathy,
Dordei, Dordi, Doretta,
Dori, Dorika, Doritha,

Dorlisa, Doro, Dorosia,
Dorota, Dorothea,
Dorothee, Dorottya,
Dorrit, Dorte, Dortha,
Dorthy, Dory, Dosi, Dossie,
Dosya, Dottie, Dotty

Drew (Greek) courageous;
strong.
Dru, Drue

Dusty (German) valiant
fighter. (English) brown
rock, quarry. A feminine
form of Dustin.
Dustee, Dusti, Dustie,
Dustina, Dustine, Dustyn

Eboni, Ebonie (Greek)
alternate forms of Ebony

Ebony (Greek) a hard,
dark wood.
Eban, Ebanee, Ebanie,
Ebany, Ebbony, Ebone,
Ebonee, Eboney, Eboni,
Ebonie, Ebonique,
Ebonisha, Ebonnee,
Ebonni, Ebonnie, Ebonye,
Ebonyi

Echo (Greek) repeated
sound. Mythology: the
nymph who pined for the

love of Narcissus until only her voice remained.
Echoe, Ekko, Ekkoe

Eden (Babylonian) a plain. (Hebrew) delightful. Bible: the earthly paradise.
Ede, Edena, Edene, Edenia, Edin, Edyn

Edith (English) rich gift.
Eadith, Eda, Ede, Edetta, Edette, Edie, Edit, Edita, Edite, Editha, Edithe, Editta, Ediva, Edyta, Edyth, Edytha, Edythe

Edna (Hebrew) rejuvenation. Mythology: the wife of Enoch, according to ancient eastern legends.
Ednah, Edneisha, Ednita

Eileen (Irish) a form of Helen. See also Aileen.
Eilean, Eilena, Eilene, Eiley, Eilidh, Eilleen, Eillen, Eilyn, Eleen, Elene

Elaine (French) a form of Helen. See also Laine.
Elain, Elaina, Elainia, Elainna, Elan, Elana, Elane, Elania, Elanie, Elanit, Elanna, Elauna, Elayn, Elayna, Elayne, Ellaine

Elana (Greek) a short form of Eleanor. See also Ilana, Lana.
Elan, Elani, Elanie

Eleanor (Greek) light. An alternate form of Helen. History: Anna Eleanor Roosevelt was a U.S. delegate to the United Nations, a writer, and the thirty-second First Lady of the U.S. See also Elana, Ella, Ellen, Lena, Nellie, Nora, Noreen.
Elana, Elanor, Elanore, Eleanora, Eleanore, Elena, Elenor, Elenorah, Elenore, Eleonor, Eleonore, Elianore, Elinor, Elinore, Elladine, Ellenor, Ellie, Elliner, Ellinor, Ellinore, Elna, Elnore, Elynor, Elynore

Elena (Greek) an alternate form of Eleanor. (Italian) a form of Helen.
Eleana, Eleen, Eleena, Elen, Elene, Eleni, Elenitsa, Elenka, Elenoa, Elenola, Elina, Ellena, Lena

Eliana (Hebrew) my God has answered me. A feminine form of Eli, Elijah.
Elianna, Elianne, Elliane, Ellianna, Ellianne, Liana, Liane

Elicia (Hebrew) an alternate form of Elisha. See also Alicia.
Ellicia

Elisa (Spanish, Italian, English) a short form of Elizabeth. See also Alisa.

Elisa *(cont.)*
Elecea, Eleesa, Elesa,
Elesia, Elisia, Elisya, Ellisa,
Ellisia, Ellissa, Ellissia,
Ellissya, Ellisya, Elysa,
Elysia, Elyssia, Elyssya,
Elysya, Lisa

Elise (French, English)
a short form of Elizabeth,
Elyse. See also Lisette.
Eilis, Eilise, Elese, Élise,
Elisee, Elisie, Elisse, Elizé,
Ellice, Ellise, Ellyce, Ellyse,
Ellyze, Elsey, Elsie, Elsy,
Elyce, Elyci, Elyse, Elyze,
Lisel, Lisl, Lison

Elisha (Greek) an alternate
form of Alisha. (Hebrew)
consecrated to God.
Eleacia, Eleasha, Elecia,
Eleesha, Eleisha, Elesha,
Eleshia, Eleticia, Elicia,
Eliscia, Elishia, Elishua,
Eliska, Elitia, Ellecia,
Ellesha, Ellexia, Ellisha,
Elsha, Elysha

Elissa, Elyssa (Greek,
English) forms of Elizabeth.
Short forms of Melissa. See
also Alisa, Alyssa.
Ellissa, Ellyssa, Ilissa, Ilyssa

Eliza (Hebrew) a short form
of Elizabeth. See also Aliza.
Elizaida, Elizalina, Elize,
Elizea

Elizabeth (Hebrew)
consecrated to God.
Bible: the mother of John
the Baptist. See also Beth,
Betsy, Betty, Elsa, Lisa,
Lisette, Liza
Eliabeth, Elisa, Elisabet,
Elisabeta, Elisabeth,
Elisabethe, Elisabetta,
Elisabette, Elise, Elisebet,
Elisheba, Elisheva, Elissa,
Eliz, Eliza, Elizabee,
Elizabet, Elizabete,
Elizaveta, Elizebeth, Ellice,
Elsabeth, Elsbet, Elsbeth,
Else, Elspet, Elspeth,
Elspie, Elsy, Elysabeth,
Elyssa, Elzbieta, Erzsébet,
Helsa, Ilizzabet, Libby,
Lusa, Yelisabeta

Ella (Greek) a short form
of Eleanor. (English) elfin;
beautiful fairy-woman.
Ellamae, Ellia, Ellie, Elly

Ellen (English) a form
of Eleanor, Helen.
Elen, Elenee, Eleny, Elin,
Elina, Elinda, Ellan, Elle,
Ellena, Ellene, Ellie, Ellin,
Ellon, Elly, Ellyn, Ellynn,
Elyn

Elsa (Hebrew) a short form of
Elizabeth. (German) noble.
Ellsa, Ellse, Ellsey, Ellsie,
Ellsy, Else, Elsie, Elsje, Elsy

Elsie (German) a familiar
form of Elsa.
Elsi, Elsy

Elyse, Elysia (Latin) sweet;
blissful. Mythology:
Elysium was the dwelling
place of happy souls.
Elise, Elysha, Ilysha, Ilysia

Emerald (French) bright
green gemstone.
Emelda, Esmeralda

Emilee, Emilie (English)
forms of Emily.
Émilie, Emméie

Emilia (Italian) a form
of Amelia, Emily.
Emalia, Emelia, Emila

Emily (Latin) flatterer.
(German) industrious.
A feminine form of Emil.
See also Amelia, Emma.
**Eimile, Em, Emaili, Emaily,
Emalia, Emalie, Emeli,
Emelia, Emelie, Emeline,
Emelita, Emely, Emilee,
Emiley, Emili, Emilia,
Emilie, Émilie, Emilienne,
Emilis, Emilka, Emillie,
Emilly, Emmalee,
Emmalou, Emmaly,
Emmélie, Emmey, Emmi,
Emmie, Emmilly, Emmy,
Emmye, Emyle**

Emma (German) a short
form of Emily. See also
Amy.
**Em, Ema, Emi, Emly,
Emmaline, Emmi, Emmie,
Emmy, Emmye**

Erica (Scandinavian) ruler
of all. (English) brave ruler.
A feminine form of Eric.
See also Ricki.
**Ericca, Ericha, Ericka,
Erika, Erikka, Errica,
Errika, Eryka, Erykka**

Erin (Irish) peace. History:
another name for Ireland.
See also Arin.
**Eran, Eren, Erena, Erene,
Ereni, Eri, Erian, Erina,
Erine, Erinetta, Erinn,
Erinna, Erinne, Eryn,
Erynn, Erynne**

Estelle (French) a form
of Esther. See also Stella.
**Essie, Estee, Estel, Estela,
Estele, Estelina, Estelita,
Estell, Estella, Estellina,
Estellita, Esthella, Estrela**

Esther (Persian) star. Bible:
the Jewish captive whom
Ahasuerus made his queen.
**Essie, Estee, Ester, Esthur,
Eszter, Eszti**

Eugenia (Greek) born to
nobility. A feminine form
of Eugene. See also Gina.
**Eugenie, Eugénie,
Eugenina, Eugina, Evgenia**

Eunice (Greek) happy;
victorious. Bible: the
mother of Saint Timothy.
**Euna, Eunique, Eunise,
Euniss**

Eva (Greek) a short form
of Evangelina. (Hebrew)
an alternate form of Eve.
See also Ava.
**Éva, Evah, Evalea, Evalee,
Evike**

Evangeline (Greek) bearer
of good news.
**Eva, Evangelia, Evangelica,
Evangelina, Evangelique**

Eve (Hebrew) life. Bible: the first woman created by God.
Eva, Evelyn, Evey, Evi, Evita, Evvie, Evvy, Evy, Evyn, Ewa, Yeva

Evelyn (English) hazelnut.
Aveline, Evaleen, Evalene, Evaline, Evalyn, Evalynn, Evalynne, Eveleen, Eveline, Evelyne, Evelynn, Evelynne, Evline, Ewalina

Evette (French) an alternate form of Yvette. See also Ivette.
Evett

Evie (Hungarian) a form of Eve.
Evi, Evicka, Evike, Evy, Ewa

F

Faith (English) faithful; fidelity. See also Faye.
Fayth, Faythe

Fallon (Irish) grandchild of the ruler.
Falan, Falen, Falin, Fallan, Fallonne, Fallyn, Falon, Falyn, Falynn, Falynne

Fannie (American) a familiar form of Frances.

Fan, Fanette, Fani, Fania, Fannee, Fanney, Fanni, Fannia, Fanny, Fanya

Farah, Farrah (English) beautiful; pleasant.
Fara, Farra, Fayre

Faren, Farren (English) wanderer.
Faran, Fare, Farin, Faron, Farrahn, Farran, Farrand, Farrin, Farron, Farryn, Farye, Faryn, Feran, Ferin, Feron, Ferran, Ferren, Ferrin, Ferron, Ferryn

Fātima (Arabic) daughter of the Prophet. History: the daughter of Muhammad.
Fatema, Fathma, Fatimah, Fatime, Fatma, Fattim

Fawn (French) young deer.
Faun, Fauna, Fawna, Fawne, Fawnia, Fawnna

Faye (French) fairy; elf. (English) an alternate form of Faith.
Fae, Fay, Fayann, Fayanna, Fayette, Fayina, Fayla, Fey, Feyla

Felecia (Latin) an alternate form of Felicia.
Flecia

Felica (Spanish) a short form of Felicia.
Falisa, Felisa, Felisca, Felissa, Feliza

Felicia (Latin) fortunate; happy. A feminine form of Felix. See also Phylicia.

**Falecia, Faleshia, Falicia,
Falleshia, Fela, Felecia,
Felica, Felice, Felicidad,
Felicie, Feliciona, Felicity,
Felicya, Felisha, Felishia,
Felisiana, Felita, Felixia,
Felizia, Felka, Fellcia,
Fellishia, Felysia, Fleasia,
Fleichia, Fleishia, Flichia**

Felisha (Latin) an alternate
form of Felicia.
**Faleisha, Falesha, Falisha,
Feleasha, Feleisha,
Felesha, Flisha**

Fiona (Irish) fair, white.
Fionna

Flora (Latin) flower. A short
form of Florence.
**Fiora, Fiore, Fiorenza,
Fleur, Flo, Flor, Florann,
Florella, Florelle, Floren,
Floria, Floriana, Florianna,
Florica, Florie, Florimel**

Florence (Latin) blooming;
flowery; prosperous.
History: Florence
Nightingale, a British
nurse, is considered
the founder of modern
nursing.
**Fiorenza, Flo, Flora,
Florance, Florencia,
Florency, Florendra,
Florentia, Florentina,
Florentyna, Florenza,
Floretta, Florette, Florie,
Florina, Florine, Floris,
Flossie**

Frances (Latin) free; from
France. A feminine form
of Francis.
**Fanny, Fran, Franca,
France, Francee, Francena,
Francesca, Francess,
Francesta, Franceta,
Francetta, Francette,
Franci, Francine, Francis,
Francise, Françoise,
Francyne, Frankie,
Frannie, Franny**

Francesca (Italian) a form
of Frances.
**Franceska, Francessca,
Francesta, Franchesca,
Francisca, Franciska,
Franciszka, Frantiska,
Franzetta, Franziska**

Franchesca (Italian)
an alternate form
of Francesca.
**Cheka, Chekka, Chesca,
Cheska, Francheca,
Francheka, Franchelle,
Franchesa, Francheska,
Franchessca, Franchesska**

Francine (French) a form
of Frances.
**Franceen, Franceine,
Franceline, Francene,
Francenia, Franci, Francin,
Francina**

Frankie (American) a famil-
iar form of Frances.
**Francka, Francki, Franka,
Frankeisha, Frankey,
Franki, Frankia, Franky**

G

Gabriela, Gabriella
(Italian) alternate forms
of Gabrielle.
Gabriala, Gabrialla,
Gabrielia, Gabriellia,
Gabrila, Gabrilla

Gabrielle (French) devoted
to God. A feminine form
of Gabriel.
Gabielle, Gabreil, Gabrial,
Gabriana, Gabriela,
Gabriele, Gabriell,
Gabriella, Gabrille,
Gabrina, Gaby, Gavriella

Gail (Hebrew) a short form
of Abigail. (English) merry,
lively.
Gael, Gaela, Gaelen,
Gaelle, Gaellen, Gaila,
Gaile, Gale, Galyn, Gayla,
Gayle

Gayle (English) an alternate
form of Gail.

Gemma (Latin, Italian)
jewel, precious stone.
Gem, Gemmey, Gemmie,
Gemmy

Gena (French) a form
of Gina. A short form
of Geneva, Genevieve.
Geanna, Geena, Geenah,
Gen, Genah, Genea, Geni,
Genia, Genice, Genie,
Genita

Geneva (French) juniper
tree. A short form of
Genevieve. Geography:
a city in Switzerland.
Geena, Gen, Gena,
Geneive, Geneve, Genever,
Genevera, Genevra,
Ginevra, Ginneva, Janeva,
Jeaneva, Jeneva

Genevieve (French, Welsh)
white wave; white phan-
tom. See also Gwendolyn.
Gen, Gena, Genaveve,
Genavieve, Genavive,
Geneva, Geneveve,
Genevie, Geneviéve,
Genevievre, Genevive,
Genna, Genovieve,
Ginette, Gineveve,
Ginevieve, Ginevive,
Guinevieve, Guinivive,
Gwenevieve, Gwenivive

Genna (English) a form
of Jenna.
Gen, Gennae, Gennay,
Genni, Gennie, Genny

Georgette (French) a form
of Georgia.
Georgeta, Georgett,
Georgetta, Georjetta

Georgia (Greek) farmer.
A feminine form of
George. Art: Georgia
O'Keeffe was an American
painter known especially

for her paintings of flowers. Geography: a southern American state; a country in Eastern Europe.
Georgene, Georgette, Georgi, Georgie, Giorgi, Giorgia

Georgina (English) a form of Georgia.
Georgena, Georgene, Georgine, Giorgina

Geraldine (German) mighty with a spear. A feminine form of Gerald. See also Dena, Jeraldine.
Geralda, Geraldina, Geraldyna, Geraldyne, Gerhardine, Geri, Gerianna, Gerianne, Gerrilee, Giralda

Geri (American) a familiar form of Geraldine. See also Jeri.
Gerri, Gerrie, Gerry

Gianna (Italian) a short form of Giovanna. See also Johana, Johnna.
Geona, Geonna, Gia, Giana, Gianella, Gianetta, Gianina, Giannella, Giannetta, Gianni, Giannina, Gianny, Gianoula

Gillian (Latin) an alternate form of Jillian.
Gila, Gilana, Gilenia, Gili, Gilian, Gill, Gilliana, Gilliane, Gilliann, Gillianna, Gillianne, Gillie, Gilly, Gillyan, Gillyane, Gillyann, Gillyanne, Gyllian, Lian

Gina (Italian) a short form of Angelina, Eugenia, Regina, Virginia.
Gena, Gin, Ginah, Ginea, Gini, Ginia

Ginger (Latin) flower; spice. A familiar form of Virginia.
Gin, Ginata, Ginja, Ginjer, Ginny

Ginny (English) a familiar form of Ginger, Virginia.
Gin, Gini, Ginney, Ginni, Ginnie, Giny

Giovanna (Italian) a form of Jane.
Giavanna, Giavonna, Giovana

Giselle (German) pledge; hostage.
Gisel, Gisela, Gisele, Giséle, Gisell, Gisella, Gissell, Gissella, Gisselle, Gizela

Gladys (Latin) small sword (Irish) princess. (Welsh) a form of Claudia. Botany: a gladiolus flower.
Glad, Gladi, Gladis, Gladiz, Gladness, Gladwys, Gwladys

Glenda (Welsh) a form of Glenna.
Glanda, Glennda, Glynda

Glenna (Irish) valley, glen.
A feminine form of Glenn.
**Glenda, Glenetta, Glenina,
Glenine, Glenn,
Glennesha, Glennie,
Glenora, Gleny, Glyn**

Gloria (Latin) glory.
History: Gloria Steinem,
a leading American
feminist, founded
Ms. magazine.
**Gloresha, Gloriah,
Glorianne, Gloribel,
Gloriela, Gloriella,
Glorielle, Gloris, Glorisha,
Glorvina, Glory**

Grace (Latin) graceful.
**Engracia, Graca, Gracea,
Graceanne, Gracey, Graci,
Gracia, Gracie, Graciela,
Graciella, Gracinha, Gracy,
Grata, Gratia, Gray,
Grayce**

Greta (German) a short
form of Gretchen,
Margaret.
**Greatal, Greatel, Greeta,
Gretal, Grete, Gretel,
Gretha, Grethal, Grethe,
Grethel, Gretta, Grette,
Grieta, Gryta, Grytta**

Gretchen (German) a form
of Margaret.
Greta, Gretchin

Guadalupe (Arabic) river
of black stones.
Guadulupe, Lupe

Gurpreet (Punjabi)
religion.

Gwen (Welsh) a short form
of Gwendolyn.
**Gwenesha, Gweness,
Gweneta, Gwenetta,
Gwenette, Gweni,
Gwenisha, Gwenita,
Gwenith, Gwenn,
Gwenna, Gwennie,
Gwenny, Gwyn**

Gwendolyn (Welsh) white
wave; white browed; new
moon. Literature: the wife
of Merlin, the magician.
See also Genevieve,
Wendy.
**Guendolen, Gwen,
Gwendalin, Gwenda,
Gwendalee, Gwendaline,
Gwendalyn, Gwendela,
Gwendolen, Gwendolene,
Gwendolin, Gwendoline,
Gwendolyne, Gwendolynn,
Gwendolynne, Gwendylan**

H

Hailey (English) an alter-
nate form of Hayley.
**Hailea, Hailee, Haili,
Hailie, Hailley, Hailly**

Haley (Scandinavian)
heroine. See also Hailey,
Hayley.
**Halee, Haleigh, Hali, Halie,
Hallie**

Hallie (Scandinavian)
an alternate form of Haley.
**Hallee, Hallei, Halley,
Halli, Hally, Hallye**

Hana (Japanese) flower.
(Arabic) happiness. (Slavic)
a form of Hannah.
**Hanan, Haneen, Hania,
Hanin, Hanita, Hanja**

Hanna (Hebrew) an alternate form of Hannah.

Hannah (Hebrew)
gracious. Bible: the mother
of Samuel. See also Ana,
Ann, Anna, Nina.
**Hana, Hanna, Hannalore,
Hanneke, Hannele, Hanni,
Hannon, Honna**

Harmony (Latin)
harmonious.
**Harmon, Harmoni,
Harmonia, Harmonie**

Harpreet (Punjabi)
devoted to God.

Harriet (French) ruler
of the household.
(English) an alternate form
of Henrietta. Literature:
Harriet Beecher Stowe
was an American writer
noted for her novel
Uncle Tom's Cabin.
**Harri, Harrie, Harriett,
Harrietta, Harriette,
Harriot, Harriott, Hattie**

Hayley (English) hay
meadow. See also Hailey,
Haley.

**Haylee, Hayli, Haylie,
Hayly**

Hazel (English) hazelnut
tree; commanding
authority.
**Hazal, Hazaline, Haze,
Hazeline, Hazell, Hazelle,
Hazen, Hazyl**

Heather (English) flower-
ing heather.
**Heath, Heatherlee,
Heatherly**

Heaven (English) place
of beauty and happiness.
Bible: where God and
angels are said to dwell.
**Heavenly, Heavin, Heavyn,
Heven**

Heidi (German) a short
form of Adelaide.
**Heida, Heide, Heidie,
Hidee, Hidi, Hiede, Hiedi**

Helen (Greek) light.
See also Aileen, Alena,
Eileen, Elaine, Eleanor,
Elena, Ellen, Nellie.
**Elana, Ena, Halina, Hela,
Hele, Helena, Helene,
Helle, Hellen, Helli, Hellin,
Hellon, Helon, Yelena**

Helena (Greek) an alternate
form of Helen.
**Halena, Halina, Helaina,
Helana, Helayna, Heleana,
Heleena, Helenna, Helina,
Hellanna, Hellenna,
Helona, Helonna**

Helene (French) a form
of Helen.
**Helaine, Helayne, Heleen,
Hèléne, Helenor, Heline,
Hellenor**

Helki (Native American)
touched.
Helkey, Helkie, Helky

Henrietta (English) ruler
of the household.
A feminine form of Henry.
**Harriet, Hattie, Hatty,
Hennrietta, Hennriette,
Henny, Henrica, Henrie,
Henrieta, Henriete,
Henriette, Henryetta,
Henya, Hetta, Hetti,
Hettie, Hetty**

Hilary, Hillary (Greek)
cheerful, merry.
**Hilaree, Hilari, Hilaria,
Hilarie, Hilery, Hiliary,
Hillaree, Hillari, Hillarie,
Hilleary, Hilleree, Hilleri,
Hillerie, Hillery, Hillianne,
Hilliary, Hillory**

Holley, Holli, Hollie
(English) alternate forms
of Holly.

Holly (English) holly tree.
**Hollee, Holley, Holli,
Hollie, Hollinda, Hollis,
Hollyann**

Hope (English) hope.
Hopey, Hopi, Hopie

I

Ida (German) hardworking.
(English) prosperous.
**Idaia, Idaleena, Idaleene,
Idalena, Idalene, Idalia,
Idalina, Idaline, Idamae,
Idania, Idarina, Idarine,
Idaya, Ide, Idelle, Idette,
Idys**

Iesha (American) a form
of Aisha.
**Ieachia, Ieaisha, Ieasha,
Ieesha, Ieeshia, Ieisha,
Ieishia, Ieshia**

Ikia (Hebrew) God is my
salvation. (Hawaiian) a
feminine form of Isaiah.
**Ikaisha, Ikea, Ikeisha,
Ikeishi, Ikeishia, Ikesha,
Ikeshia**

Ilana (Hebrew) tree.
**Ilane, Ilani, Ilainie, Illana,
Illane, Illani, Ilania,
Illanie, Ilanit**

India (Hindi) from India.
Indi, Indie, Indy, Indya

Ingrid (Scandinavian)
hero's daughter; beautiful
daughter.
Inga, Inge, Inger

Irene (Greek) peaceful.
Mythology: the goddess
of peace. See also Rena,
Rene.
**Eirena, Erena, Ira, Irana,
Iranda, Iranna, Irén,
Irena, Irenea, Irenka,
Iriana, Irien, Irina, Jereni**

Iris (Greek) rainbow.
Mythology: the goddess
of the rainbow and
messenger of the gods.
Irisa, Irisha, Irissa, Irita

Isabel (Spanish) conse-
crated to God. A form
of Elizabeth.
**Isa, Isabal, Isabeau,
Isabela, Isabeli, Isabelita,
Isabella, Ishbel, Isobel,
Issi, Issie, Issy, Iza, Izabel,
Izabele**

Isabelle (French) a form
of Isabel.
Isabella, Izabelle

Ivette (French) an alternate
form of Yvette. See also
Evette.
**Ivete, Iveth, Ivetha, Ivetta,
Ivey**

Ivory (Latin) made of ivory.
Ivori, Ivorine, Ivree

Ivy (English) ivy tree.
Ivey, Ivie

J

Jacalyn (American) a form
of Jacqueline.
**Jacelyn, Jacelyne, Jacelynn,
Jacilyn, Jacilyne, Jacilynn,
Jacolyn, Jacolyne,
Jacolynn, Jacylyn,
Jacylyne, Jacylynn**

Jacey (Greek) a familiar
form of Jacinda.
(American) a combination
of the initials J. + C.
**Jace, Jac-E, Jacee, Jacia,
Jacie, Jaciel, Jacy, Jacylin**

Jacinda, Jacinta (Greek)
beautiful, attractive.
**Jacenda, Jacenta, Jacey,
Jacinth, Jacintha, Jacinthe,
Jacynth, Jakinda, Jaxine**

Jacki, Jackie (American)
familiar forms of
Jacqueline.
**Jackee, Jackia, Jackielee,
Jacky**

Jacklyn (American) a short
form of Jacqueline.
**Jacklin, Jackline, Jacklyne,
Jacklynn, Jacklynne**

Jackqueline (French) an
alternate form of
Jacqueline.

Jackqueline (cont.)
Jackquelin, Jackquilin,
Jackquiline

Jaclyn (American) a short
form of Jacqueline.
Jacleen, Jaclin, Jacline,
Jaclyne, Jaclynn

Jacqueline (French)
supplanter, substitute;
little Jacqui. A feminine
form of Jacques.
Jacalyn, Jackalyn, Jackie,
Jacklyn, Jaclyn, Jacqualin,
Jacqualine, Jacqualyn,
Jacqualyne, Jacqualynn,
Jacqueleen, Jacquelene,
Jacquelin, Jacquelyn,
Jacquelynn, Jacqui,
Jacquil, Jacquilin,
Jacquiline, Jacquilyn,
Jacquilyne, Jacquilynn,
Jacquine, Jaquelin,
Jaqueline, Jaquelyn,
Jaquelyne, Jaquelynn,
Jockeline, Jocqueline

Jacquelyn, Jacquelynn
(French) alternate forms
of Jacqueline.
Jacquelyne

Jade (Spanish) jade.
Jada, Jadah, Jadda, Jadea,
Jadeann, Jadee, Jaden,
Jadera, Jadi, Jadie,
Jadielyn, Jadienne, Jady,
Jadzia, Jadziah, Jaeda,
Jaedra, Jaida, Jaide, Jaiden

Jaime (French) I love.
Jaima, Jaimee, Jaimey,
Jaimi, Jaimini, Jaimmie,
Jaimy

Jaimee (French) an alternate form of Jaime.

Jami, Jamie (Hebrew)
supplanter, substitute.
(English) feminine forms
of James.
Jama, Jamay, Jamea,
Jamee, Jameka, Jamesha,
Jamia, Jamielee, Jamiesha,
Jamii, Jamika, Jamilynn,
Jamis, Jamise, Jammie,
Jamy, Jamya, Jamye,
Jayme, Jaymee, Jaymie

Jamila (Arabic) beautiful.
Jahmela, Jahmelia, Jahmil,
Jahmilla, Jamee, Jameela,
Jameelah, Jameeliah,
Jameila, Jamela, Jamelia,
Jameliah, Jamell, Jamella,
Jamelle, Jamely, Jamelya,
Jamiela, Jamilah, Jamilee,
Jamilia, Jamiliah, Jamilla,
Jamillah, Jamille, Jamillia,
Jamilya, Jamyla, Jemeela,
Jemelia, Jemila, Jemilla

Jamilynn (English) a com-
bination of Jami + Lynn.
Jamielin, Jamieline,
Jamielyn, Jamielyne,
Jamielynn, Jamielynne,
Jamilin, Jamiline, Jamilyn,
Jamilyne, Jamilynne

Jammie (American) a form
of Jami.

Jammesha, Jammi, Jammice, Jammise, Jammisha

Jan (English) a short form of Jane, Janet, Janice.
Jani, Jania, Jandy, Jannie

Jana (Slavic) a form of Jane.
Janaca, Janalee, Janalisa, Janalynn, Janika, Janka, Janna, Janne

Janae, Janay (American) forms of Jane.
Janaé, Janaea, Janaeh, Janah, Janai, Janaya, Janaye, Janea, Janee, Janée, Jannae, Jannay, Jenae, Jenay, Jenaya, Jennae, Jennay, Jennaya, Jennaye

Jane (Hebrew) God is gracious. A feminine form of John. See also Giovanna, Jean, Joan, Juanita, Shauna, Shawna, Sheena.
Jaine, Jan, Jana, Janae, Janay, Janean, Janeann, Janelle, Janen, Janene, Jannessa, Janet, Jania, Janice, Janie, Janika, Janine, Janique, Janis, Janka, Janna, Jannie, Jasia, Jayna, Jayne, Jenica, Jenny, Joanna, Joanne, Sinead

Janel, Janell (French) alternate forms of Janelle.
Jannel, Jaynel, Jaynell

Janelle (French) a form of Jane.

Janel, Janela, Janele, Janelis, Janell, Janella, Janelli, Janellie, Janelly, Janely, Janelys, Janiel, Janielle, Janille, Jannel, Jannell, Jannelle, Jannellies, Janyll, Jaynelle

Janessa (American) a form of Jane.
Janesha, Janeska, Janiesa, Janiesha, Janisha, Janissa, Jannesa, Jannesha, Jannessa, Jannisa, Jannisha, Jannissa

Janet (English) a form of Jane. See also Jessie.
Jan, Janeta, Janete, Janett, Janetta, Janette, Janita, Janith, Janitza, Jannet, Janneta, Janneth, Jannetta, Jannette, Janot, Jante, Janyte

Janice (Hebrew) God is gracious. (English) a familiar form of Jane.
Jan, Janece, Janecia, Janeice, Janiece, Janika, Janitza, Janizzette, Jannice, Janniece, Jannika, Janyce, Jynice

Janie (English) a familiar form of Jane.
Janey, Jani, Jany

Janine (French) a form of Jane.
Janeen, Janenan, Janene, Janina, Jannina, Jannine, Jannyne, Janyne, Jenine

Janis (English) a form
of Jane.
**Janees, Janeesa, Janesa,
Janese, Janesey, Janesia,
Janessa, Janesse, Janise,
Janisha, Janissa, Jannis,
Jannisa, Jannisha,
Jannissa, Jenesa, Jenessa,
Jenesse, Jenice, Jenis,
Jenisha, Jenissa, Jennisa,
Jennise, Jennisha,
Jennissa, Jennisse**

Janna (Hebrew) a short
form of Johana. (Arabic)
harvest of fruit.
Janaya, Janaye

Jasmine (Persian) jasmine
flower. See also Yasmin.
**Jas, Jasma, Jasmain,
Jasmaine, Jasman, Jasme,
Jasmeen, Jasmeet,
Jasmene, Jasmin, Jasmina,
Jasmira, Jasmit, Jasmon,
Jasmyn, Jassma, Jassmain,
Jassmaine, Jassmin,
Jassmine, Jassmit,
Jassmon, Jassmyn, Jazmin**

Jaspreet (Punjabi) virtuous.
**Jas, Jaspar, Jasparit,
Jasparita, Jasper, Jasprit,
Jasprita, Jasprite**

Jaye (Latin) jaybird.
Jae, Jay, Jaylene

Jaylene (American) a form
of Jaye.
**Jayelene, Jayla, Jaylah,
Jaylan, Jayleana, Jaylee,
Jayleen**

Jayme, Jaymie (English)
alternate forms of Jami.
**Jaymi, Jaymia, Jaymine,
Jaymini**

Jayna (Hebrew) an alternate form of Jane.
Jaynae

Jayne (Hindi) victorious.
(English) a form of Jane.
**Jayn, Jaynee, Jayni, Jaynie,
Jaynita, Jaynne**

Jazmin, Jazmine (Persian)
alternate forms of Jasmine.
**Jazman, Jazmen, Jazminn,
Jazmon, Jazmyn, Jazmyne,
Jazzman, Jazzmen,
Jazzmin, Jazzmine,
Jazzmit, Jazzmon,
Jazzmyn**

Jean, Jeanne (Scottish)
God is gracious. Forms
of Jane, Joan.
**Jeana, Jeanann, Jeancie,
Jeane, Jeaneane, Jeaneen,
Jeaneia, Jeanell, Jeanelle,
Jeanette, Jeaneva, Jeanice,
Jeanie, Jeanine, Jeanmarie,
Jeanna, Jeanné, Jeannee,
Jeanney, Jeannie, Jeannita,
Jeannot, Jeanny, Jeantelle**

Jeana, Jeanna (Scottish)
alternate forms of Jean.

Jeanette (French) a form
of Jean.
**Jeanete, Jeanett,
Jeanetta, Jeanita,
Jeannete, Jeannett,
Jeannetta, Jeannette,
Jeannita, Jenet, Jenett,**

Jenette, Jennet, Jennett,
Jennetta, Jennette,
Jennita, Jinetta, Jinette

Jeanie (Scottish) a familiar
form of Jean.
Jeani, Jeanny, Jeany

Jeanine, Jenine (Scottish)
alternate forms of Jean.
Jeanene, Jeanina,
Jeannina, Jeannine,
Jennine

Jena (Arabic) an alternate
form of Jenna.
Jenae, Jenah, Jenai, Jenal,
Jenay

Jenelle (American) a com-
bination of Jenny + Nell.
Jenall, Jenalle, Jenel,
Jenell, Jenille, Jennel,
Jennell, Jennelle, Jennielle,
Jennille

Jenifer, Jeniffer (Welsh)
alternate forms of Jennifer.

Jenilee (American) a com-
bination of Jenni + Lee.
Jenalea, Jenalee,
Jenaleigh, Jenaly, Jenelea,
Jenelee, Jeneleigh, Jenely,
Jenelly, Jenileigh, Jenily,
Jennely, Jennielee,
Jennilea, Jennilee, Jennilie

Jenna (Arabic) small bird.
(Welsh) a short form of
Jennifer. See also Genna.
Jena, Jennah, Jennat,
Jennay, Jhenna

Jenni, Jennie (Welsh)
familiar forms of Jennifer.

Jeni, Jenica, Jenisa, Jenka,
Jenne, Jenné, Jennee,
Jenney, Jennia, Jennier,
Jennita, Jennora, Jensine

Jennica (Romanian) a form
of Jane.
Jenica, Jenika, Jennika

Jennifer (Welsh) white
wave; white phantom.
Jen, Jenefer, Jenifer,
Jeniffer, Jenipher, Jenna,
Jennafer, Jenniferanne,
Jenniferlee, Jenniffe,
Jenniffer, Jenniffier,
Jennifier, Jennilee,
Jenniphe, Jennipher,
Jenny, Jennyfer

Jenny (Welsh) a familiar
form of Jennifer.
Jenney, Jenni, Jennie, Jeny,
Jinny

Jeraldine (English) a form
of Geraldine.
Jeraldeen, Jeraldene,
Jeraldina, Jeraldyne,
Jeralee, Jeri

Jeri, Jerri, Jerrie
(American) short forms
of Jeraldine.
Jera, Jerae, JeRae, Jeree,
Jeriel, Jerilee, Jerilyn,
Jerina, Jerinda, Jerra,
Jerrece, Jerriann, Jerrilee,
Jerrine, Jerry, Jerrylee,
Jerryne, Jerzy

Jerica (American) a combination of Jeri + Erica.

Jerica *(cont.)*
**Jerice, Jericka, Jerika,
Jerreka, Jerrica, Jerricca,
Jerrice, Jerricka, Jerrika**

Jerilyn (American) a combi-
nation of Jeri + Lynn.
**Jeralin, Jeraline, Jeralyn,
Jeralyne, Jeralynn,
Jeralynne, Jerelin, Jereline,
Jerelyn, Jerelyne, Jerelynn,
Jerelynne, Jerilin, Jeriline,
Jerilyne, Jerilynn,
Jerilynne, Jerrilin,
Jerriline, Jerrilyn,
Jerrilyne, Jerrilynn,
Jerrilynne**

Jessalyn (American) a com-
bination of Jessica + Lynn.
**Jesalin, Jesaline, Jesalyn,
Jesalyne, Jesalynn,
Jesalynne, Jesilin, Jesiline,
Jesilyn, Jesilyne, Jesilynn,
Jesilynne, Jessalin,
Jessaline, Jessalyne,
Jessalynn, Jessalynne,
Jesselin, Jesseline,
Jesselyn, Jesselyne,
Jesselynn, Jesselynne**

Jesse, Jessi (Hebrew) alternate forms of Jessie.
Jessey

Jessenia (Arabic) flower.
Jescenia, Jesenia

Jessica (Hebrew) wealthy.
A feminine form of Jesse.
Literature: a name perhaps
invented by Shakespeare
for a character in his play
The Merchant of Venice.

**Jesi, Jesica, Jesika, Jess,
Jessa, Jessaca, Jessah,
Jessalyn, Jessca, Jesscia,
Jesseca, Jessia, Jessicca,
Jessicia, Jessicka, Jessie,
Jessieka, Jessika, Jessiqua,
Jessiya, Jessy, Jessyca,
Jessyka, Jezeca, Jezica,
Jezika, Jezyca**

Jessie (Hebrew) a short
form of Jessica. (Scottish)
a form of Janet.
**Jescie, Jesey, Jess, Jesse,
Jessé, Jessee, Jessi, Jessia,
Jessiya, Jessy, Jessye**

Jessika (Hebrew) an alternate form of Jessica.

Jill (English) a short form
of Jillian.
**Jil, Jiline, Jilli, Jillie, Jilline,
Jillisa, Jillissa, Jilly, Jillyn**

Jillian (Latin) youthful.
An alternate form of Julia.
See also Gillian.
**Jilian, Jiliana, Jiliann,
Jilianna, Jilianne, Jilienna,
Jilienne, Jill, Jillaine,
Jilliana, Jilliane, Jilliann,
Jillianne, Jillien, Jillienne,
Jillion, Jilliyn**

Jo (American) a short form
of Joanna, Jolene,
Josephine.
**Joangie, Joetta, Joette,
Joey**

Joan (Hebrew) God is gracious. An alternate form
of Jane. History: Joan of
Arc was a fifteenth-century

heroine and resistance
fighter. See also Jean,
Juanita, Siobhan.
**Joane, Joaneil, Joanel,
Joanelle, Joanie,
Joanmarie, Joann,
Joannanette, Joannel**

Joanie (Hebrew) a familiar
form of Joan.
**Joani, Joanni, Joannie,
Joany, Joenie, Joni**

Joanna (English) a form
of Joan.
**Janka, Jo, Joana, Jo-Ana,
Joandra, Joanka,
Joananna, Joananne,
Jo-Anie, Joanka, Jo-Anna,
Joannah, Jo-Annie, Joayn,
Joeana, Joeanna, Johana,
Johanna, Johannah**

Joanne (English) a form
of Joan.
**Joanann, Joananne, Joann,
Jo-Ann, Jo-Anne, Joeann,
Joeanne**

Jocelyn (Latin) joyous.
**Jocelin, Joceline, Jocelle,
Jocelyne, Jocelynn,
Jocelynne, Joci, Jocia,
Jocinta, Joscelin, Jossalin,
Josilin, Joycelyn**

Jodi, Jodie, Jody
(American) familiar forms
of Judith.
**Jodee, Jodele, Jodell,
Jodelle, Jodene, Jodevea,
Jodilee, Jodi-Lee, Jodilynn,
Jodi-Lynn, Jodine, Jodyne**

Joelle (Hebrew) God is
willing. A feminine form
of Joel.
**Joel, Joela, Joelee, Joeleen,
Joelene, Joeli, Joeline,
Joell, Joella, Joëlle, Joellen,
Joelly, Joellyn, Joelyn,
Joelyne, Joelynn**

Johana, Johanna
(German) forms of Joanna.
**Janna, Johanah, Johani,
Johanie, Johanka,
Johannah, Johanne,
Johanni, Johannie, Johnna,
Johonna, Jonna**

Johnna, Jonna (American)
forms of Joanna, Johana.
See also Gianna.
**Jahna, Jahnaya, Jhona,
Jhonna, Jianna, Jianni,
Jiannini, Johna, Johnda,
Johneatha, Johnetta,
Johnette, Johni, Johnica,
Johnie, Johnique, Johnita,
Johnittia, Johnnessa,
Johnni, Johnnie,
Johnnielynn, Johnnie-
Lynn, Johnnquia, Johnny,
Johnquita, Joncie, Jonda,
Jondell, Jondrea, Jonni,
Jonnica, Jonnie, Jonnika,
Jonnita, Jonny, Jonyelle,
Jutta**

Joleen, Joline (English)
alternate forms of Jolene.

Jolene (Hebrew) God will
add, God will increase.
(English) a form of
Josephine.

Jolene (cont.)
Jo, Jolaine, Jolana, Jolane, Jolanna, Jolanne, Jolanta, Jolayne, Jole, Jolean, Joleane, Jolee, Joleen, Jolena, Joléne, Jolenna, Joley, Jolin, Jolina, Jolinda, Joline, Jolinna, Jolisa, Jolleane, Jolleen, Jollene, Jolline, Jolye

Jonelle (American) a combination of Joan + Elle.
Jahnel, Jahnell, Jahnelle, Johnel, Johnell, Johnella, Johnelle, Jonel, Jonell, Jonella, Jynell, Jynelle

Joni (American) a familiar form of Joan.
Jona, Jonae, Jonai, Jonann, Jonati, Joncey, Jonci, Joncie, Joneeka, Joneen, Joneika, Joneisha, Jonelle, Jonessa, Jonetia, Jonetta, Jonette, Jonica, Jonice, Jonie, Jonika, Jonilee, Jonilee, Jonina, Joniqua, Jonique, Jonis, Jonisa, Jonisha, Jonit, Jony

Jordan (Hebrew) descending.
Jordain, Jordana, Jordane, Jordanna, Jorden, Jordenne, Jordi, Jordin, Jordine, Jordon, Jordonna, Jordyn, Jordyne, Jori, Jorie

Jordana, Jordanna
(Hebrew) alternate forms of Jordan.

Jordann, Jordanne, Jourdana, Jourdann, Jourdanna, Jourdanne

Josee, Josée (American) familiar forms of Josephine.
Joesee, Joesell, Joesette, Joselle, Josette, Josey, Josi, Josiane, Josiann, Josianne, Josielina, Josina, Josy, Jozee, Jozelle, Jozette, Jozie

Joselyn, Joslyn (Latin) alternate forms of Jocelyn.
Josalene, Joselene, Joseline, Josiline, Josilyn

Josephine (French) God will add, God will increase. A feminine form of Joseph.
Fina, Jo, Joey, Josee, Josée, Josefa, Josefena, Josefina, Josefine, Josepha, Josephe, Josephene, Josephin, Josephina, Josephyna, Josephyne, Josette, Josie, Sefa

Josie (Hebrew) a familiar form of Josephine.
Josee, Josey, Josi, Josy, Josye

Joslyn (Latin) an alternate form of Jocelyn.
Josielina, Josiline, Josilyn, Josilyne, Josilynn, Josilynne, Joslin, Josline, Joslyne, Joslynn, Joslynne

Joy (Latin) joyous.
Joi, Joie, Joya, Joyan, Joyann, Joyanna,

**Joyanne, Joye, Joyeeta,
Joyelle, Joyhanna,
Joyhannah, Joyia, Joylin,
Joyline, Joylyn, Joylyne,
Joylynn, Joylynne, Joyous,
Joyvina**

Joyce (Latin) joyous.
A short form of Jocelyn.
**Joice, Joycey, Joycie,
Joyous, Joysel**

Juanita (Spanish) a form
of Jane, Joan.
**Juana, Juandalyn,
Juaneice, Juanequa,
Juanesha, Juanice,
Juanicia, Juaniqua,
Juanisha, Juanishia,
Juanna**

Judith (Hebrew) praised.
Mythology: the slayer
of Holofernes, according
to ancient eastern legend.
**Giuditta, Ioudith, Jodi,
Jodie, Jody, Jucika, Judana,
Jude, Judine, Judit, Judita,
Judite, Juditha, Judithe,
Judy, Judyta, Jutka**

Judy (Hebrew) a familiar
form of Judith.
Juci, Judi, Judie, Judye

Julia (Latin) youthful.
A feminine form of Julius.
See also Jill, Jillian.
**Iulia, Jula, Julene, Juliana,
Juliann, Julica, Julie, Juliet,
Julija, Julina, Juline, Julisa,
Julissa, Julita, Julyssa**

Juliana (Czech, Spanish),
Julianna (Hungarian)
forms of Julia.
Julliana, Jullianna

Juliann, Julianne (English)
forms of Julia.
**Juliane, Julieann,
Julie-Ann, Julieanne,
Julie-Anne**

Julie (English) a form
of Julia.
**Juel, Jule, Julee, Juli,
Julie-Lynn, Julie-Mae,
Julien, Juliene, Julienne,
Jullie, July**

Juliet, Juliette (French)
forms of Julia.
**Julet, Julieta, Julietta,
Jullet, Julliet, Jullietta**

June (Latin) born in the
sixth month.
**Juna, Junell, Junelle,
Junette, Junia, Junie,
Juniet, Junieta, Junietta,
Juniette, Junina, Junita**

Justina (Italian) a form
of Justine.
**Jestena, Jestina, Justinna,
Justyna**

Justine (Latin) just,
righteous. A feminine
form of Justin.
**Giustina, Jestine, Juste,
Justi, Justie, Justina,
Justinn, Justy, Justyne**

K

Kacey, Kacy (Irish) brave.
(American) alternate forms
of Casey. A combination
of the initials K. + C.
**K. C., Kace, Kacee, Kaci,
Kacie, Kaicee, Kaicey,
Kasey, Kasie, Kaycee,
Kayci, Kaycie**

Kaci, Kacie (American)
alternate forms of Kacey,
Kacy.
Kasci, Kaycie, Kaysie

Kady (English) an alternate
form of Katy. A combina-
tion of the initials K. + D.
**Cady, K. D., Kade, Kadee,
Kadey, Kadi, Kadie, Kayde,
Kaydee, Kaydey, Kaydi,
Kaydie, Kaydy**

Kaela (Hebrew, Arabic)
beloved sweetheart.
**Kaelah, Kayla, Kaylah,
Keyla, Keylah, Kaelyn**

Kaelyn (American) a com-
bination of Kaela + Lynn.
See also Kaylyn.
**Kaelan, Kaelen, Kaelin,
Kaelinn, Kaelynn,
Kaelynne**

Kaila (Hebrew) laurel;
crown.

**Kailah, Kailee, Kailey,
Kayla**

Kailee, Kailey (American)
familiar forms of Kaila.
Alternate forms of Kayley.
Kaile, Kaili

Kaitlin (Irish) pure. An
alternate form of Caitlin.
See also Katelin.
**Kaitlan, Kaitland,
Kaitleen, Kaitlen, Kaitlind,
Kaitlinn, Kaitlon, Kalyn**

Kaitlyn (Irish) an alternate
form of Caitlyn.
Kaitlynn, Kaitlynne

Kala (Arabic) beloved,
sweetheart.
Kalila

Kaleena (Hawaiian) pure.
Kalena, Kalina

Kaley (American) an alter-
nate form of Caleigh,
Caley, Kayley.
Kalee, Kaleigh, Kalleigh

Kali (Sanskrit) energy;
black goddess; time the
destroyer. (Hawaiian)
hesitating. Religion:
a name for the Hindu
goddess Shakti. See
also Cali.
**Kala, Kalee, Kaleigh,
Kaley, Kalie, Kallee, Kalley,
Kalli, Kallie, Kally, Kallye,
Kaly**

Kalli, Kallie (Greek) an
alternate form of Callie.

**Kalle, Kallee, Kalley,
Kallita, Kally**

Kalyn (American) an alternate form of Kaylyn.

Kami (Italian, North African) a short form of Kamila, Kamilah. (Japanese) divine aura. See also Cami.
Kammi, Kammie, Kammy, Kamy

Kandace, Kandice (Greek) glittering white; glowing. (American) alternate forms of Candace, Candice.
Kandas, Kandess, Kandi, Kandis, Kandise, Kandiss, Kandus, Kandyce, Kandys, Kandyse

Kara (Greek, Danish) pure. An alternate form of Katherine.
Kaira, Kairah, Karah, Karalea, Karaleah, Karalee, Karalie, Kari

Karah (Greek, Danish) an alternate form of Kara. (Irish, Italian) an alternate form of Cara.
Karrah

Karen (Greek) pure. An alternate form of Katherine. See also Carey, Carina, Caryn.
Kaaren, Kaarin, Kaarina, Kalina, Karaina, Karan, Karena, Karin, Karina, Karine, Karna, Karon, Karren, Karrin, Karrina,

Karrine, Karron, Karyn, Kerrin, Kerron, Kerrynn, Kerrynne, Koren

Kari (Greek) pure. (Danish) a form of Caroline, Katherine. See also Carey, Cari, Carrie.
Karee, Karey, Kariann, Karianna, Karianne, Karle, Karrey, Karri, Karrie, Karry, Kary

Karin (Scandinavian) a form of Karen.
Karina, Karine, Karinne

Karina (Russian) a form of Karen.
Karinna, Karrina, Karryna, Karyna

Karine (Russian) a form of Karen.
Karrine, Karryne, Karyne

Karissa (Greek) an alternate form of Carissa.
Karese, Karessa, Karesse, Karisa, Karisha, Karishma, Karisma, Karissimia, Kariza, Karrisa, Karrissa, Karyssa

Karla (German) an alternate form of Carla.
Karila, Karilla, Karle, Karleen, Karleigh, Karlen, Karlena, Karlene, Karlenn, Karletta, Karley, Karlicka, Karlign, Karlin, Karlina, Karling, Karlinka, Karlisha, Karlisia, Karlita, Karlitha, Karla, Karlon,

Karla *(cont.)*
Karlyan, Karlye, Karlyn, Karlynn, Karlynne

Karli, Karly (Latin) little and womanly. (American) forms of Carly.
Karlee, Karley, Karlie, Karlye

Karmen (Hebrew) song. A form of Carmen.
Karman, Karmencita, Karmin, Karmina, Karmine, Karmita, Karmon, Karmyn, Karmyne

Karolyn (American) a form of Carolyn.
Karalyn, Karalyna, Karalynn, Karalynne, Karilyn, Karilyna, Karilynn, Karilynne, Karlyn, Karlynn, Karlynne, Karolyna, Karolynn, Karolynne, Karrolyn, Karrolyna, Karrolynn, Karrolynne

Karri, Karrie (American) forms of Carrie.
Kari, Karie, Karry

Karyn (American) a form of Karen.
Karyna, Karyne, Karynn

Kasey, Kasie (Irish) brave. (American) forms of Casey, Kacey.
Kaisee, Kaisie, Kasci, Kascy, Kasee, Kasi, Kasy, Kasya, Kaysci, Kaysea, Kaysee, Kaysey, Kaysi, Kaysie, Kaysy

Kasi (Hindi) from the holy city.

Kassandra (Greek) an alternate form of Cassandra.
Kasander, Kasandria, Kasandra, Kasaundra, Kasondra, Kasoundra, Kassandr, Kassandre, Kassandré, Kassaundra, Kassi, Kazandra, Khrisandra, Krisandra, Krissandra

Kassi, Kassie (American) familiar forms of Kassandra, Kassidy. See also Cassie.
Kassey, Kassia, Kassy

Kassidy (Irish) clever. (American) an alternate form of Cassidy.
Kassadee, Kassadi, Kassadie, Kassadina, Kassady, Kasseday, Kassedee, Kassi, Kassiddy, Kassidee, Kassidi, Kassidie, Kassity

Katarina (Czech) a form of Katherine.
Kata, Katarin, Kataryna, Katerina, Katerine, Katerini, Katrika, Katrina, Katrine

Kate (Greek) pure. (English) a short form of Katherine.
Kait, Kata, Kati, Katica, Katja, Katy, Katya

Katelin, Katelyn (Irish)
alternate forms of Caitlin.
See also Kaitlin.
Kaetlin, Kaetlyn,
Kaetlynn, Kaetlynne,
Katalin, Katelan,
Kateland, Kateleen,
Katelen, Katelene,
Katelind, Katelinn,
Katelun, Katelynn, Katlyn,
Kaytlin, Kaytlyn,
Kaytlynn, Kaytlynne

Katharine (Greek) an alter-
nate form of Katherine.
Katharaine, Katharin,
Katharina, Katharyn

Katherine (Greek) pure.
See also Carey, Catherine,
Kara, Karen, Kari.
Ekaterina, Ekatrinna,
Kasienka, Kasin, Kat,
Katarina, Katchen, Kate,
Katha, Kathann,
Kathanne, Katharine,
Kathereen, Katheren,
Katherene, Katherenne,
Katherin, Katherina,
Katheryn, Katheryne,
Kathi, Kathleen, Kathryn,
Kathy, Kathyrine, Katina,
Katlaina, Katoka,
Katreeka, Katrina, Kay,
Kitty

Kathi, Kathy (English)
familiar forms of
Katherine, Kathleen.
See also Cathi.
Kaethe, Katha, Kathe,
Kathee, Kathey, Kathi,
Kathie, Katla, Kató

Kathleen (Irish) a form
of Katherine. See also
Cathleen.
Katheleen, Kathelene,
Kathileen, Kathlyn,
Kathlyne, Kathlynn,
Kathy, Katleen, Katlin,
Katlyn, Katlynn

Kathrine (English) a form
of Katherine.
Kathren, Kathryn,
Kathryne

Katlyn (Greek) pure.
(Irish) an alternate form
of Katelin.
Kaatlain, Katland, Katlin,
Katlynd, Katlynn,
Katlynne

Katrina (German) a form
of Katherine. See also
Catrina, Trina.
Katina, Katja, Katreen,
Katreena, Katrelle,
Katrene, Katri, Katrice,
Katricia, Katrien, Katrin,
Katrine, Katrinia,
Katriona, Katryn,
Katryna, Kattiah,
Kattrina, Kattryna, Katya

Katy (English) a familiar
form of Kate.
Kady, Katey, Katya, Kayte

Kay (Greek) rejoicer.
(Teutonic) a fortified place.
(Latin) merry. A short form
of Katherine.
Caye, Kae, Kai, Kaye,
Kayla

Kaycee (American) a combination of the initials
K. + C.

Kayla (Arabic, Hebrew)
laurel; crown. An alternate
form of Kaela, Kaila.
Kaela, Kaila, Kayle,
Kaylee, Kayleen, Kaylene,
Kaylia, Kaylin

Kayleen, Kaylene
(Hebrew) beloved,
sweetheart. Alternate
forms of Kayla.
Kaeleen, Kaelen, Kaelene,
Kailen, Kaileen, Kailene,
Kaylen

Kayleigh (American) an
alternate form of Kayley.
Kaeleigh, Kaileigh

Kayley, Kaylie (American)
forms of Kayla.
Caeley, Kaelea, Kaeleah,
Kaelee, Kaeli, Kaelie,
Kaelee, Kaeli, Kaelie,
Kailea, Kaileah, Kailee,
Kayle, Kaylea, Kayleah,
Kaylee, Kaylei, Kayleigh,
Kayley, Kayli

Kaylin (American) an alternate form of Kaylyn.
Kaylan, Kaylon

Kaylyn (American) a com-
bination of Kay + Lynn.
See also Kaelyn.
Kailyn, Kailynn, Kailynne,
Kayleen, Kaylene,
Kaylynn, Kaylynne

Keara (Irish) dark; black.
Religion: an Irish saint.
Kearia, Kearra, Keera,
Keerra, Keira, Keirra,
Kera, Kiara, Kiarra, Kiera,
Kierra

Keeley, Keely (Irish) alter-
nate forms of Kelly.
Kealee, Kealey, Keali,
Kealie, Keallie, Kealy,
Kealyn, Keela, Keelan,
Keelee, Keeleigh, Keeli,
Keelie, Keelin, Keellie,
Keelyn, Keighla, Keilan,
Keilee, Keileigh, Keiley,
Keilly, Kiela, Kiele, Kieley,
Kielly, Kiely, Kielyn

Keena (Irish) brave.
Keenya, Kina

Keira (Irish) an alternate
form of Kiara.
Kera

Keisha (American) a form
of Aisha.
Keesha, Keishaun,
Keishauna, Keishawn,
Kesha, Keysha, Kiesha,
Kisha, Kishanda

Kelley (Irish) an alternate
form of Kelly.

Kelli, Kellie (Irish) familiar
forms of Kelly.
Keli, Kelia, Kellia,
Kelliann, Kellianne, Kellisa

Kelly (Irish) brave warrior.
See also Caleigh.

Keeley, Keely, Kelley, Kellyann, Kellyanne, Kelley, Kelli, Kellie, Kellye

Kellyn (Irish) a combination of Kelly + Lyn.
Kelleen, Kellen, Kellene, Kellina, Kelline, Kellynn, Kellynne

Kelsey (Scandinavian, Scottish) ship island. (English) an alternate form of Chelsey.
Kelcey, Kelcy, Kelda, Kellsee, Kellsei, Kellsey, Kellsie, Kellsy, Kelsa, Kelsea, Kelsei, Kelsey, Kelsi, Kelsie, Kelsy, Keslie

Kelsi, Kelsie (Scottish) forms of Chelsea.
Kelci, Kelcie

Kendall (English) ruler of the valley.
Kendahl, Kendal, Kendalla, Kendalle, Kendel, Kendele, Kendell, Kendelle, Kendera, Kendia, Kendyl, Kendyle, Kendyll, Kinda, Kindal, Kindall, Kindi, Kindle, Kynda, Kyndal, Kyndall

Kendra (English) water baby. (Dakota) magical power.
Kendre, Kenna, Kenndra, Kentra, Kentrae, Kindra, Kyndra

Kenna (Irish) beautiful. A feminine form of Kenneth.
Kennia

Kenya (Hebrew) animal horn. Geography: a country in Africa.
Keenya, Kenia, Kenja

Kenzie (Scottish) light skinned. (Irish) a short form of Mackenzie.
Kenzy, Kinzie

Kera (Irish) a short form of Kerry.

Keren (Hebrew) animal's horn.
Kerrin, Keryn

Kerri, Kerrie (Irish) alternate forms of Kerry.
Keri, Keriann, Kerianne, Kerriann, Kerrianne

Kerry (Irish) dark haired. Geography: a county in Ireland.
Keree, Kerey, Kerri, Kerrie, Kerryann, Kerryanne, Kiera, Kierra

Keshia (American) an alternate form of Keisha.
Kecia, Keishia, Keschia, Kesha, Kesia, Kesiah, Kessiah

Khadijah (Arabic) trustworthy. History: Muhammed's first wife.
Khadeeja, Khadeja, Khadjha, Khadija

Kia (African) season's beginning. (American) a short form of Kiana.
Kiah

Kiana (American) a combination of the prefix Ki + Ana.
Keanna, Keiana, Kiani, Kiahna, Kianna, Kianni, Kiauna, Kiandra, Kiandria, Kiauna, Kiaundra, Kiona, Kionah, Kioni, Kionna

Kiara (Irish) little and dark. A feminine form of Kieran.

Kiera, Kierra (Irish) alternate forms of Kerry.
Kierana, Kieranna, Kierea

Kiley (Irish) attractive; from the straits.
Kilee, Kilie, Kylee, Kyli, Kylie

Kim (Vietnamese) needle. (English) a short form of Kimberly.
Kimba, Kimbra, Kimee, Kimette, Kimme, Kimmee, Kimmi, Kimmie, Kimmy, Kimy, Kym

Kimberlee, Kimberley (English) alternate forms of Kimberly.
Kimbalee, Kimberlea, Kimberlei, Kimberleigh, Kimbley

Kimberly (English) chief, ruler.
Cymbre, Kim, Kimba, Kimbely, Kimber, Kimbereley, Kimberely, Kimberlee, Kimberli, Kimberlie, Kimberlyn, Kimbery, Kimbria,

Kimbrie, Kimbry, Kymberly

Kinsey (English) offspring; relative.
Kinsee

Kira (Persian) sun. (Latin) light. A feminine form of Cyrus.
Kiran, Kirby, Kiri, Kiria

Kirsta (Scandinavian) an alternate form of Kirsten.

Kirsten (Greek) Christian; annointed. (Scandinavian) a form of Christine.
Karsten, Keirstan, Kerstin, Kiersten, Kirsteni, Kirsta, Kirstan, Kirsteen, Kirstene, Kirstin, Kirston, Kirsty, Kirstyn, Kjersten, Kursten, Kyrsten

Kirstin (Scandinavian) an alternate form of Kirsten.
Karstin, Kirstien, Kirstine

Kita (Japanese) north.

Kori (American) a form of Corey.
Koree, Korey, Koria, Korie, Korri, Korrie, Korry, Kory

Kortney (English) an alternate form of Courtney.
Kortnay, Kortnee, Kortni, Kortnie, Kortny

Kourtney (American) a form of Courtney.
Kourtni, Kourtny, Kourtynie

Krista (Czech) a form of Christina. See also Christa.
Khrissa, Khrista, Khryssa, Khrysta, Krissa, Kryssa, Krysta

Kristen (Greek) Christian; annointed. (Scandinavian) a form of Christine.
Christen, Kristan, Kristin, Krysten

Kristi, Kristie (Scandinavian) short forms of Kristine.
Christi

Kristian, Kristiana (Greek) Christian; anointed. Alternate forms of Christian.
Khristian, Kristian, Kristiann, Kristi-Ann, Kristianna, Kristianne, Kristi-Anne, Kristien, Kristienne, Kristiin, Kristyan, Kristyana, Kristy-Ann, Kristy-Anne

Kristin (Scandinavian) an alternate form of Kristen. See also Cristen.
Kristyn, Krystin

Kristina (Greek) Christian; annointed. (Scandinavian) a form of Christina. See also Cristina.
Khristina, Kristina, Kristeena, Kristena, Kristiana, Kristianna, Krysteena, Krystena, Krystiana, Krystianna, Krystina, Krystyna

Kristine (Scandinavian) a form of Christine.
Kristeen, Kristene, Kristi, Kristiane, Kristie, Kristy, Kristyn, Krystine, Krystyne

Kristy (American) a familiar form of Kristine, Krystal. See also Cristy.
Kristi, Kristia, Kristie, Krysia, Krysti

Krysta (Polish) a form of Krista.
Krystka

Krystal (American) clear, brilliant glass. A form of Crystal.
Kristabel, Kristal, Kristale, Kristall, Kristel, Kristell, Kristelle, Kristill, Kristl, Kristle, Kristy, Krystalann, Krystalanne, Krystale, Krystaleen, Krystalina, Krystall, Krystel, Krystelle, Krystil, Krystle, Krystol

Krystina (Czech) a form of Kristin.
Krysten, Krystin, Krystyna

Krystle (American) an alternate form of Krystal.
Krystl, Krystyl

Kyla (Irish) attractive. (Yiddish) crown; laurel.
Kylen, Kylene, Kylia, Kylynn

Kyle (Irish) attractive.
Kial, Kiele, Kylee, Kylene,
Kylie

Kylee (Irish) a familiar form
of Kyle.
Kylea, Kyleah, Kyleigh,
Kylie

Kylene (Irish) an alternate
form of Kyle.
Kylen, Kylyn

Kylie (West Australian
Aboriginal) curled stick;
boomerang. (Irish)
a familiar form of Kyle.
Keiley, Keilley, Keilly,
Keily, Kiley, Kye, Kylee

Kymberly (English)
an alternate form
of Kimberly.
Kymberlee, Kymberley,
Kymberlie, Kymberlyn

Kyra (Greek) ladylike.
Keera, Keira, Kira, Kyrah,
Kyrene, Kyria, Kyriah,
Kyriann, Kyrie

L

Lacey, Lacy (Greek)
a familiar form of Larissa.
(Latin) cheerful.
Lacee, Laci, Lacie

Ladonna (American)
a combination of the
prefix La + Donna.
Ladon, Ladona, Ladonne,
Ladonya

Laila (Arabic) an alternate
form of Leila.
Laili, Lailie

Laine (French) a short form
of Elaine.
Laina, Lainee, Lainey,
Layney

Lakeisha (American)
a combination of the
prefix La + Keisha.
Lakaiesha, Lakaisha,
Lakasha, Lakecia,
Lakeesh, Lakeesha,
Lakesha, Lakeshia,
Lakeshya, Lakesia,
Laketia, Lakeysha,
Lakeyshia, Lakezia,
Lakicia, Lakiesha,
Lakieshia, Lakisha,
Lakitia

Lakendra (American)
a combination of the
prefix La + Kendra.
Lakanda, Lakedra

**Lakesha, Lakeshia,
Lakisha** (American) alter-
nate forms of Lakeisha.
Lakecia, Lakeesha,
Lakeseia, Lakiesha

Lakia (Arabic) found
treasure.
Lakita

Lana (Latin) woolly.
(Irish) attractive, peaceful.
A short form of Alana,
Elana. (Hawaiian) floating;
bouyant.
**Lanae, Lanata, Lanay,
Laneetra, Lanette, Lanna,
Lannah, Lanny**

Lani (Hawaiian) sky;
heaven. A short form of
Leilani.
Lanita, Lannie

Laquisha (American)
a combination of the
prefix La + Queisha.
**Laquasha, Laquaysha,
Laqueisha, Laquesha,
Laquiesha**

Laquita (American)
a combination of the
prefix La + Quintana.
**Laqeita, Laqueta,
Laquetta, Laquia,
Laquiata, Laquinta,
Laquitta**

Lara (Greek) cheerful.
(Latin) shining; famous.
Mythology: the daughter
of the river god Almo.
A short form of Larissa,
Laura.
Larah, Laretta, Larette

Larissa (Greek) cheerful.
See also Lacey.
Laris, Larisa, Laryssa

Lashanda (American)
a combination of the
prefix La + Shanda.
**Lashana, Lashanay,
Lashandra, Lashane,
Lashanna, Lashannon,
Lashanta, Lashante**

Lashawna (American)
a combination of the
prefix La + Shawna.
**Lashaun, Lashauna,
Lashaune, Lashaunna,
Lashaunta, Lashawn,
Lashawnd, Lashawnda,
Lashawndra, Lashawne,
Lashawnia, Leshawn,
Leshawna**

Lashonda (American)
a combination of the
prefix La + Shonda.
**Lachonda, Lashaunda,
Lashaundra, Lashon,
Lashona, Lashond,
Lashonde, Lashondia,
Lashondra, Lashonna,
Lashonta, Lashunda,
Lashundra, Lashunta,
Lashunte, Leshande,
Leshandra, Leshondra,
Leshundra**

Latanya (American)
a combination of the
prefix La + Tanya.
**Latana, Latandra, Latania,
Latanja, Latanna,
Latanua, Latona, Latoni,
Latonia, Latonna,
Latonshia, Latonya**

Latara (American)
a combination of the
prefix La + Tara.

Latasha (American)
a combination of the
prefix La + Tasha.
**Latacha, Latacia, Latai,
Lataisha, Latashia,
Lataysha, Letasha,
Letashia, Leteshia,
Letasiah, Leteisha**

Latavia (American) a combination of the prefix La +
Tavia.

Latesha (American) a form
of Leticia.
**Lataeasha, Lateashia,
Latecia, Lateesha,
Lateicia, Lateisha, Latesa,
Lateshia, Latessa, Latisa,
Latissa**

Latia (American)
a combination of the
prefix La + Tia.
Latea, Lateia, Lateka

Latisha (Latin) joy. An
alternate form of Leticia.
**Laetitia, Laetizia,
Latashia, Latia, Latice,
Laticia, Lateasha,
Lateashia, Latecia,
Lateesha, Lateicia,
Lateisha, Lateshia,
Latiesha, Latishia,
Latissha, Latitia**

Latonya (American) a
combination of the prefix
La + Tonya.
Latoni, Latonia, Latonna

Latoria (American)
a combination of the
prefix La + Tori.

**Latorio, Latorja, Latorray,
Latorreia, Latory, Latorya,
Latoyra, Latoyria**

Latosha (American)
a combination of the
prefix La + Tosha.
Latoshia, Latosia

Latoya (American)
a combination of the
prefix La + Toya.
**Latoia, Latoira, Latoiya,
LaToya, Latoyia, Latoye,
Latoyia, Latoyita, Latoyo,
Latoyra, Latoyria**

Latrice (American)
a combination of the
prefix La + Trice.
**Latrece, Latreece,
Latreese, Latresa, Latrese,
Latressa, Letreece, Letrice**

Latricia (American)
a combination of the
prefix La + Tricia.
**Latrecia, Latresh,
Latresha, Latreshia,
Latrica, Latrisha, Latrishia**

Laura (Latin) crowned
with laurel. A feminine
form of Laurence.
**Lara, Lauralee,
Laureana, Laurel,
Laurelen, Laurella,
Lauren, Lauriana,
Lauriane, Lauricia, Laurie,
Laurina, Laurka, Lavra,
Lolly, Lora, Loretta, Lori,
Lorinda, Lorina, Lorinda,
Lorita, Lorna, Loura**

Laurel (Latin) laurel tree.
**Laural, Laurell, Laurelle,
Lorel, Lorelle**

Lauren (English) a form
of Laura.
**Laureen, Laurena,
Laurene, Laurin, Lauryn,
Laurynn, Loren**

Laurie (English) a familiar
form of Laura.
**Lari, Larilia, Laure, Lauré,
Lauri, Lawrie, Lori**

Lawanda (American)
a combination of the
prefix La + Wanda.
Lawynda

Layla (Hebrew, Arabic)
an alternate form of Leila.
Layli, Laylie

Lea (Hawaiian) Mythology:
the goddess of canoe
makers.

Leah (Hebrew) weary.
Bible: the wife of Jacob.
See also Lia.
**Lea, Léa, Lee, Leea, Leeah,
Leia, Leigh**

Lean, Leanne (English)
forms of Leeann.
**Leana, Leane, Leann,
Leanna**

Leandra (Latin) like
a lioness.
**Leanda, Leandre,
Leandrea, Leandria,
Leeanda, Leeandra**

Lee (Chinese) plum.
(Irish) poetic. (English)
meadow. A short form
of Ashley, Leah.
Lea, Leigh

Leeann, Leeanne
(English) a combination
of Lee + Ann.
**Leane, Leanna, Leean,
Leeanna, Leian, Leiann,
Leianna, Leianne**

Leigh (English) an alternate
form of Lee.
**Leigha, Leighann,
Leighanna, Leighanne**

Leila (Hebrew) dark beauty;
night. (Arabic) born at
night. Literature: the heroine of the epic Persian
poem *Leila and Majnum*.
See also Layla, Lila.
**Laila, Layla, Leela, Leelah,
Leilah, Leilia, Lela, Lelah,
Leland, Lelia, Leyla**

Leilani (Hawaiian) heavenly
flower; heavenly child.
Lani, Lei, Lelani, Lelania

Lena (Greek) a short
form of Eleanor. (Hebrew)
dwelling or lodging.
(Latin) temptress.
(Norwegian) illustrious.
Music: Lena Horne,
a well-known African
American singer.
**Lenah, Lene, Lenea,
Lenee, Lenette, Leni,
Lenka, Lina, Linah**

Leona (German) brave as a lioness. A feminine form of Leon.
Leoine, Leola, Leolah, Leone, Leonelle, Leonia, Leonice, Leonicia, Léonie, Leonine, Leonissa, Liona

Lesley (Scottish) gray fortress.
Leslea, Leslee, Leslie, Leslye, Lezlee, Lezley, Lezli, Lezly

Leslie (Scottish) an alternate form of Lesley.
Lesli, Lesslie

Leticia (Latin) joy. See also Latesha, Latisha, Tisha.
Leisha, Leshia, Let, Leta, Letha, Lethia, Letice, Letichia, Letisha, Letisia, Letita, Letitia, Letiza, Letizia, Letty, Letycia, Loutitia

Lia (Greek) bringer of good news. (Hebrew, Dutch, Italian) dependent. See also Leah.
Liah

Liana (Hebrew) a short form of Eliana. (Latin) youth. (French) bound, wrapped up; tree covered with vines. (English) meadow.
Leanna, Liane, Lianna, Lianne

Liane, Lianne (Hebrew) alternate forms of Liana.

Liberty (Latin) free.

Lidia (Greek) an alternate form of Lydia.
Lidi, Lidka, Lyda

Lila (Arabic) night. (Hindi) free will of god. (Persian) lilac. A short form of Delilah, Lillian.
Lilah, Lilia, Lyla, Lylah

Lillian (Latin) lily flower.
Lian, Lil, Lila, Lilas, Lileana, Lileane, Lilia, Lilian, Liliana, Liliane, Lilias, Liliha, Lilja, Lilla, Lilli, Lillia, Lillianne, Lis, Liuka

Lily (Latin, Arabic) a familiar form of Lillian.
Lil, Líle, Lili, Lilie, Lilijana, Lilika, Lilike, Liliosa, Lilium, Lilka, Lille, Lilli, Lillie, Lilly

Lina (Greek) light. (Latin) an alternate form of Lena (Arabic) tender.
Lin

Linda (Spanish) pretty.
Lin, Lind, Lindee, Lindey, Lindi, Lindie, Lindy, Linita, Lynda

Lindsay (English) an alternate form of Lindsey.
Lin, Lindsi, Lyndsay, Lyndsaye, Linsay

Lindsey (English) linden tree island; camp near the stream.

Lin, Lind, Lindsea, Lindsee, Lindsi, Linsey, Lyndsey, Lynsey

Lindsi (American) a familiar form of Lindsay, Lindsey.
Lin, Lindsie, Lindsy, Lindzy

Linette, Lynnette (Welsh) idol. (French) bird.
Lanette, Lin, Linet, Linnet, Linnetta, Linnette, Lynette, Lynnet

Linnea (Scandinavian) lime tree. History: the national flower of Sweden.
Lin, Linea, Linnaea, Lynea, Lynnea

Linsey (English) an alternate form of Lindsey.
Lin, Linsi, Linsie, Linsy, Linzee, Linzey, Linzi, Linzy, Lynsey

Lisa (Hebrew) consecrated to God. (English) a short form of Elizabeth.
Leesa, Leeza, Liesa, Liisa, Lisa-Marie, Lisanne, Lise, Lisette, Litsa, Liza, Lysa

Lise (German) a form of Lisa.

Lisette (French) a form of Lisa. (English) a familiar form of Elise, Elizabeth.
Liseta, Lisetta, Lisettina, Lissette

Liza (American) a short form of Elizabeth.
Leeza, Liz, Lizete, Lizette, Lizka, Lizzie, Lyza

Lois (German) famous warrior. An alternate form of Louise.

Lola (Spanish) a familiar form of Dolores, Louise.
Lolita

Loni (English) solitary.
Lonee, Lonie, Lonni, Lonnie

Lora (Latin) crowned with laurel. (American) a form of Laura.
Lorah, Lorane, Lorann, Lorra, Lorrah, Lorrane

Loren (American) an alternate form of Lauren.
Loreen, Lorena, Lorin, Lorine, Lorne, Lorren, Lorrin, Lorryn, Loryn, Lorynn, Lorynne

Lorena (English) an alternate form of Lauren, Loren.
Loreen, Lorene, Lorenia, Lorenna, Lorrina, Lorrine

Loretta (English) a familiar form of Laura.
Larretta, Lauretta, Laurette, Loretah, Lorette, Lorita, Lorretta, Lorrette

Lori (Latin) crowned with laurel. (French) a short form of Lorraine. (American) a familiar form of Laura.
Laurie, Loree, Lorey, Loria, Lorianna, Lorianne, Lorie, Lorree, Lorrie, Lory

Lorna (Latin) crowned with laurel. An alternate form of Laura. Literature: probably coined by Richard Blackmore in his novel *Lorna Doone*.
Lorrna

Lorraine (Latin) sorrowful. (French) from Lorraine. See also Rayna.
Laraine, Lauraine, Laurraine, Lorain, Loraine, Lorayne, Lorein, Loreine, Lori, Lorine, Lorrain, Lorraina, Lorrayne, Lorreine

Louisa (English) a familiar form of Louise. Literature: Louisa May Alcott was an American writer and reformer best known for her novel *Little Women*.
Aloisa, Eloisa, Heloisa, Lou, Louisian, Louisane, Louisina, Louiza, Lovisa, Ludovica, Ludovika, Ludwiga, Luisa, Luiza, Lujza, Lujzika, Lula, Lulita

Louise (German) famous warrior. A feminine form of Louis. See also Alison, Lois, Lola.
Loise, Lou, Louisa, Louisette, Louisiane, Louisine, Lourdes, Lowise, Loyce, Loyise, Lu, Luisa, Luise

Lucia (Italian, Spanish) a form of Lucy.
Luciana, Lucianna

Lucie (French) a familiar form of Lucy.

Lucille (English) a familiar form of Lucy.
Lucila, Lucile, Lucilla

Lucinda (Latin) a familiar form of Lucy. See also Cindy.
Lucka, Lucky

Lucy (Latin) light; bringer of light.
Lou, Lu, Luca, Luce, Lucetta, Luci, Lucia, Lucida, Lucie, Lucienne, Lucille, Lucinda, Lucine, Lucita, Luciya, Lucya, Luzca, Luz, Luzi

Luisa (Spanish) a form of Louisa.

Luz (Spanish) light. Religion: Santa Maria de Luz is another name for the Virgin Mary.
Luzi, Luzija

Lydia (Greek) from Lydia, an ancient land once ruled by Midas. (Arabic) strife.
Lida, Lidi, Lidia, Lidija, Lidiya, Lyda, Lydie, Lydië

Lynda (Spanish) pretty. (American) a form of Linda.
Lyndall, Lynde, Lyndee, Lyndi, Lyndy, Lynnda, Lynndie, Lynndy

Lyndsay (American) a form of Lindsay.

Lyndsey (English) linden tree island; camp near the stream. (American) a form of Lindsey.
Lyndsea, Lyndsee, Lyndsi, Lyndsie, Lyndsy, Lynndsie

Lynette (Welsh) idol. (English) a form of Linette.
Lynett, Lynetta, Lynnette

Lynn, Lynne (English) waterfall; pool below a waterfall.
Lin, Lina, Linn, Lyn, Lyndel, Lyndell, Lyndella, Lynette, Lynlee, Lynley, Lynna, Lynnell

Lynsey (American) an alternate form of Lyndsey.
Lynnsey, Lynnzey, Lynsie, Lynsy, Lynzey, Lynzi, Lynzie, Lynzy

M

Mabel (Latin) lovable.
Mab, Mabelle, Mable, Mabyn, Maible, Maybel, Maybelle, Maybull

Mackenzie (Irish) daughter of the wise leader. See also Kenzie.
Macenzie, Mackensi, Mackensie, Mackenzee, Mackenzi, Mackenzia, Mackenzy, McKenzie, Mekenzie, Mykenzie

Madeleine (French) a form of Madeline.
Madelaine, Madelayne

Madeline (Greek) high tower. (English) from Magdala, England. See also Lena, Lina.
Mada, Madailéin, Madalaina, Madaleine, Madalena, Madaline, Maddalena, Maddie, Madel, Madeleine, Madelena, Madelene, Madelia, Madelina, Madella, Madelle, Madelon, Madelyn, Madge, Madlen, Madlin, Madline, Madoline, Magdalen, Maida, Malena

Madelyn (Greek) an alternate form of Madeline.
Madalyn, Madalynn, Madalynne, Madelynn, Madelynne, Madlyn, Madolyn

Madison (English) good; son of Maud.
Madisen, Madissen, Madisyn, Madysen, Madyson

Maegan (Irish) an alternate form of Megan.
Maeghan

Magan, Magen (Greek) short forms of Margaret.

Magdalena (Greek) high tower. Bible: Magdala was the home of Saint Mary Magdalen. See also Madeline, Marlene.
Mada, Magda, Magdala, Magdalen, Magdalene, Magdalina, Magdaline, Magdalyn, Magdelana, Magdelane, Magdelene, Magdelina, Magdeline, Magdelyn, Magdlen, Magdolna, Maggie, Magola, Mahda, Maighdlin, Makda, Mala, Malaine, Maudlin

Maggie (Greek) pearl. (English) a familiar form of Magdalena, Margaret.
Mag, Magge, Maggee, Maggen, Maggey, Maggi, Maggia, Maggiemae, Maggin, Maggy, Mags

Maia (Greek) mother; nurse. (English) kinswoman; maiden. Mythology: the loveliest of the Pleiades, the seven daughters of Atlas, and the mother of Hermes. See also Maya.
Maiah, Maie, Maya, Mayam, Mya

Makayla (American) an alternate form of Michaela.
Mikayla

Malia (Hawaiian, Zuni) a form of Mary. (Spanish) a form of Maria

Malea, Maleah, Maleia, Maliaka, Maliasha, Malie, Maliea, Malli, Mally

Malika (Hungarian) industrious.
Maleeka, Maleka, Mali

Malinda (Greek) an alternate form of Melinda.
Malinde, Malinna, Malynda

Malissa (Greek) an alternate form of Melissa.

Mallorie (French) an alternate form of Mallory.

Mallory (German) army counselor. (French) unlucky.
Malerie, Maliri, Mallari, Mallary, Mallauri, Mallerie, Mallery, Malley, Malloree, Malloreigh, Mallorey, Mallori, Mallorie, Malori, Malorie, Malory, Malorym, Malree, Malrie, Mellory, Melorie, Melory

Mandeep (Punjabi) enlightened.

Mandis (Xhosa) sweet.

Mandy (Latin) lovable. A familiar form of Amanda, Melinda.
Mandee, Mandi, Mandie

Manpreet (Punjabi) mind full of love.

Mara (Greek) eternally beautiful. (Slavic) a form of Mary.
Mahra, Marah, Maralina, Maraline, Marra

Maranda (Latin) an alternate form of Miranda.

Marcella (Latin) martial, warlike. Mythology: Mars was the god of war.
Mairsil, Marca, Marce, Marceil, Marcela, Marcele, Marcelen, Marcelia, Marcell, Marcelle, Marcello, Marcena, Marchella, Marchelle, Marci, Marcie, Marciella, Marcile, Marcilla, Marcille, Marcy, Marella, Marsella, Marselle, Marsiella

Marci, Marcie (English) familiar forms of Marcella, Marcia.
Marcee, Marcita, Marcy, Marsi, Marsie

Marcia (Latin) martial, warlike. An alternate form of Marcella. See also Marquita.
Marcena, Marchia, Marci, Marciale, Marcie, Marcsa, Marsha, Martia

Marcy (English) an alternate form of Marci.
Marsey, Marsy

Maren (Latin) sea. (Aramaic) a form of Mary. See also Marina.

Marena, Marin, Marina, Miren, Mirena

Margaret (Greek) pearl. History: Margaret Hilda Thatcher served as British prime minister. See also Greta, Gretchen, Marjorie, Markita, Megan, Peggy.
Madge, Maergrethe, Magan, Magen, Maggie, Maisie, Mamie, Maretta, Marga, Margalit, Margalith, Marganit, Maretha, Margarett, Margaretta, Margarette, Margarid, Margarida, Margaro, Margaux, Marge, Margeret, Margeretta, Margerette, Margerie, Margerite, Marget, Margetta, Margette, Margie, Margisia, Margit, Margo, Margot, Margret, Marguerite, Meta

Margarita (Italian, Spanish) a form of Margaret. See also Rita.
Margareta, Margarit, Margaritis, Margaritt, Margaritta, Margharita, Margherita, Margrieta, Margrita, Marguarita, Marguerita, Margurita

Margie (English) a familiar form of Margaret.
Margey, Margi, Margy

Margo, Margot (French) forms of Margaret.
Mago, Margaro

Marguerite (French)
a form of Margaret.
**Margarete, Margaretha,
Margarethe, Margarite,
Margerite, Marguaretta,
Marguarette, Marguarite,
Marguerette, Margurite**

Mari (Japanese) ball.
(Spanish) a form of Mary.

Maria (Hebrew) bitter;
sea of bitterness. (Italian,
Spanish) a form of Mary.
**Maie, Malia, Marea,
Mareah, Maree,
Mariabella, Mariae, Marie,
Mariesa, Mariessa,
Mariha, Marija, Mariya,
Marja, Marya**

Mariah (Hebrew)
an alternate form of
Mary. See also Moriah.
**Maraia, Maraya, Mariyah,
Marriah, Meriah**

Mariam (Hebrew) an alter-
nate form of Miriam.
**Maryam, Mariem,
Meryam**

Marian (English) an alter-
nate form of Maryann.
**Mariana, Mariane,
Mariann, Marianne,
Mariene, Marion, Marrian,
Marriann, Marrianne,
Maryann, Maryanne**

Mariana (Spanish) a form
of Marian.
**Marianna, Marriana,
Marrianna, Maryana,
Maryanna**

Maribel (French) beautiful.
(English) a combination
of Maria + Bell.
**Marabel, Marbelle,
Mariabella, Maribella,
Maribelle, Maridel,
Marybel, Marybella,
Marybelle**

Marie (French) a form
of Mary.
**Manon, Maree, Marie-
Claude, Marie-Eve, Marie-
Pier, Marietta, Marrie**

Mariel (German, Dutch)
a form of Mary.
**Marial, Marieke, Mariela,
Mariele, Marieline,
Mariella, Marielle,
Mariellen, Marielsie,
Mariely, Marielys**

Marika (Dutch, Slavic)
a form of Mary.
**Marica, Marieke, Marija,
Marijke, Marike, Marikia,
Mariska, Mariske,
Marrika, Maryk, Maryka,
Merica, Merika**

Marilyn (Hebrew) Mary's
line or descendants.
**Maralin, Maralyn,
Maralyne, Maralynn,
Maralynne, Marelyn,
Marilin, Marillyn,
Marilynn, Marilynne,
Marlyn, Marolyn,
Marralynn, Marrilin,
Marrilyn, Marrilynn,
Marrilynne, Marylin,
Marylinn, Marylyn,**

Marylyne, Marylynn, Marylynne

Marina (Latin) sea. See also Maren, Marnie.
Marena, Marenka, Marinda, Marindi, Marine, Marinka, Marrina, Maryna, Merina

Marion (French) a form of Mary.
Marrian, Marrion, Maryon, Maryonn

Marisa (Latin) sea.
Mariesa, Mariessa, Marisela, Marissa, Marita, Mariza, Marrisa, Marrissa, Marysa, Maryse, Maryssa, Merisa

Marisela (Latin) an alternate form of Marisa.
Mariseli, Marisella, Marishelle

Marisha (Russian) a familiar form of Mary.
Marishenka, Marishka, Mariska

Marisol (Spanish) sunny sea.
Marise, Marizol

Marissa (Latin) an alternate form of Marisa.
Maressa, Marisa, Marisha, Marisse, Marrissa, Marrissia, Merissa, Morissa

Maritza (Arabic) blessed

Marjorie (Greek) a familiar form of Margaret. (Scottish) a form of Mary.
Majorie, Marge, Margeree, Margerey, Margerie, Margery, Margorie, Margory, Marjarie, Marjary, Marjerie, Marjery, Marjie, Marjorey, Marjori, Marjory

Markita (Czech) a form of Margaret.
Marka, Markeda, Markee, Markeeta, Marketa, Marketta, Markia, Markie, Markieta, Markita, Markitha, Markketta

Marla (English) a short form of Marlena, Marlene.
Marlah, Marlea, Marleah

Marlana (English) a form of Marlena.
Marlania, Marlanna

Marlee (English) a form of Marlene.
Marlea, Marleah

Marlena (German) a form of Marlene.
Marla, Marlaina, Marlana, Marlanna, Marleena, Marlina, Marlinda, Marlyna, Marna

Marlene (Greek) high tower. (Slavic) a form of Magdalena.
Marla, Marlaine, Marlane, Marlayne, Marlee, Marleen, Marlena,

Marlene (cont.)
**Marlenne, Marley,
Marline, Marlyne**

Marley (English) a familiar
form of Marlene.
**Marlee, Marli, Marlie,
Marly**

Marnie (Hebrew) a short
form of Marina.
**Marna, Marne, Marnee,
Marney, Marni, Marnja,
Marnya**

Marquita (Spanish) a form
of Marcia.
**Marqueda, Marquedia,
Marquee, Marqueita,
Marquet, Marqueta,
Marquetta, Marquette,
Marquia, Marquida,
Marquietta, Marquitra,
Marquitia, Marquitta**

Marsha (English) a form
of Marcia.
**Marcha, Marshae,
Marshay, Marshayly,
Marshel, Marshele,
Marshell, Marshia,
Marshiela**

Marta (English) a short
form of Martha, Martina.
**Martá, Martä, Martaha,
Marte, Marttaha, Merta**

Martha (Aramaic) lady;
sorrowful. Bible: a sister
of the Virgin Mary.
**Maita, Marta, Martaha,
Marth, Marthan, Marthe,
Marthena, Marthina,
Marthine, Marthy, Marti,**

**Marticka, Martita, Matti,
Mattie, Matty, Martus,
Martuska, Masia**

Martina (Latin) martial,
warlike. A feminine form
of Martin. See also Tina.
**Marta, Martel, Martella,
Martelle, Martene,
Marthena, Marthina,
Marthine, Marti, Martine,
Martinia, Martino,
Martisha, Martiza,
Martosia, Martoya,
Martricia, Martrina,
Martyna, Martyne,
Martynne**

Mary (Hebrew) bitter; sea
of bitterness. An alternate
form of Miriam. Bible: the
mother of Jesus. See also
Malia, Maren, Mariah,
Marjorie, Maura, Maureen,
Miriam, Moira, Molly,
Muriel.
**Maire, Manette, Manka,
Manon, Manya, Mara,
Marabel, Mare, Maree,
Maren, Marella, Marelle,
Mari, Maria, Mariam,
Marian, Maricara, Marice,
Maridel, Marie, Mariel,
Marika, Marilee, Marilla,
Marilyn, Marion,
Mariquilla, Mariquita,
Marisha, Marita, Marité,
Maritsa, Maritza, Marja,
Marjan, Marje, Marlo,
Maroula, Maruca, Marye,
Maryla, Marynia, Maryse,
Marysia, Masha, Maurise,**

**Maurizia, Mavra, Mendi,
Mérane, Meridel, Merrili,
Mhairie, Mirja, Mirjam,
Molara, Morag, Moya,
Muire**

Maryann, Maryanne
(English) combinations
of Mary + Ann.
**Mariann, Marianne,
Maryanna**

Marybeth (American)
a combination of
Mary + Beth.
Maribeth, Maribette

Mattie, Matty (English)
familiar forms of Martha
**Matte, Mattey, Matti,
Mattye**

Maura (Irish) dark. An
alternate form of Mary,
Maureen. See also Moira.
**Maure, Maurette,
Mauricette, Maurita**

Maureen (French) dark.
(Irish) a form of Mary.
**Maura, Maurene,
Maurine, Mo, Moreen,
Morena, Morene, Morine,
Morreen, Moureen**

Maxine (Latin) greatest.
A feminine form of
Maximillian.
**Max, Maxa, Maxeen,
Maxena, Maxene, Maxi,
Maxie, Maxima, Maxime,
Maximiliane, Maxina,
Maxna, Maxy, Maxyne**

May (Latin) great. (Arabic)
discerning. (English)
flower; month of May.
**Mae, Maj, Maybelle,
Mayberry, Maybeth,
Mayday, Maydee,
Maydena, Maye, Mayela,
Mayella, Mayetta,
Mayrene**

Maya (Hindi) God's creative
power. (Greek) mother;
grandmother. (Latin)
great. An alternate form
of Maia.

McKenzie (Scottish) a form
of Mackenzie.
**McKenna, McKensi,
McKinzie**

Mead, Meade (Greek)
honey wine.

Meagan (Irish) an alternate
form of Megan.
**Maegan, Meagain,
Meagann, Meagen,
Meagin, Meagnah,
Meagon**

Meaghan (Welsh) a form
of Megan.
**Maeghan, Meaghann,
Meaghen, Meahgan**

Megan (Greek) pearl;
great. (Irish) a form
of Margaret.
**Maegan, Magan, Meagan,
Meaghan, Magen, Meg,
Megean, Megen, Meggan,
Meggen, Meghan, Megyn,
Meygan**

Meghan (Welsh) a form
of Megan.
Meeghan, Meehan,
Megha, Meghana,
Meghane, Meghann,
Meghanne, Meghean,
Meghen, Mehgan,
Mehgen

Meka (Hebrew) a familiar
form of Michaela.

Melanie (Greek) dark
skinned.
Malania, Malanie, Meila,
Meilani, Meilin, Meladia,
Melaine, Melainie,
Melana, Melane, Melanee,
Melaney, Melani, Melania,
Mélanie, Melanney,
Melannie, Melantha,
Melany, Melanya, Melasya,
Melayne, Melenia, Melina,
Mella, Mellanie, Melonie,
Melya, Melyn, Melyne,
Melynn, Melynne, Milana,
Milena, Milya

Melina (Latin) canary
yellow. (Greek) a short
form of Melinda.
Melaina, Meleana,
Meleena, Melena, Meline,
Melinia, Melinna, Melynna

Melinda (Greek) honey.
See also Linda, Melina,
Mindy.
Maillie, Malinda, Melinde,
Melinder, Mellinda,
Melynda, Milinda,
Milynda, Mylinda,
Mylynda

Melissa (Greek) honey bee.
See also Elissa, Millicent.
Malissa, Mallissa,
Melesa, Melessa, Meleta,
Melisa, Mélisa, Melise,
Melisha, Melishia, Melisia,
Mélissa, Melisse, Melissia,
Meliza, Melizah, Mellie,
Mellisa, Mellissa, Melly,
Melosa, Milisa, Milissa,
Millie, Milly, Misha, Missy,
Molissia, Mollissa, Mylisa,
Mylisia, Mylissa, Mylissia

Melody (Greek) melody.
Melodee, Melodey,
Melodi, Melodia, Melodie,
Melodye

Melonie (American) an
alternate form of Melanie.
Melloney, Mellonie,
Mellony, Melonee,
Meloney, Meloni,
Melonnie, Melony

Mercedes (Latin) reward,
payment. (Spanish)
merciful.
Merced, Mercede,
Mersade

Meredith (Welsh) protec-
tor of the sea.
Meredithe, Meredy,
Meredyth, Meredythe,
Meridath, Merideth,
Meridie, Meridith,
Merridie, Merridith,
Merry

Meryl (German) famous.
(Irish) shining sea. An
alternate form of Muriel.

Meral, Merel, Merrall,
Merrell, Merril, Merrill,
Merryl, Meryle, Meryll

Mia (Italian) mine. A familiar form of Michaela,
Michelle.
Mea, Meah, Miah

Micah (Hebrew) a short form of Michaela. Bible: one of the Old Testament prophets.
Mica, Mika, Myca, Mycah

Michaela (Hebrew) who is like God? A feminine form of Michael.
Machaela, Makayla, Meecah, Mia, Micaela, Michael, Michaelann, Michealia, Michaelina, Michaeline, Michaell, Michaella, Michaelle, Michaelyn, Michaila, Michal, Michala, Micheal, Micheala, Michela, Michelia, Michelina, Michelle, Michely, Michelyn, Micheyla, Micheline, Micki, Micquel, Miguela, Mikaela, Miquel, Miquela, Miquelle, Mycala, Mychael, Mychal

Michele (Italian) a form of Michaela.
Michela

Michelle (French) who is like God? A form of Michaela. See also Shelley.
Machealle, Machele, Machell, Machella,

Machelle, Mechelle, Meichelle, Meschell, Meshell, Meshelle, Mia, Michel, Michele, Michèle, Michell, Michella, Michellene, Michellyn, Mischel, Mischelle, Misha, Mishae, Mishael, Mishaela, Mishayla, Mishell, Mishelle, Mitchele, Mitchelle

Mika (Hebrew) an alternate form of Micah. (Russian) God's child. (Native American) wise racoon.
Mikah

Mikaela (Hebrew) an alternate form of Michaela.
Mekaela, Mekala, Mekayla, Mickael, Mickaela, Mickala, Mickalla, Mickayla, Mickeel, Mickell, Mickelle, Mikail, Mikaila, Mikal, Mikalene, Mikalovna, Mikalyn, Mikayla, Mikayle, Mikea, Mikeisha, Mikeita, Mikel, Mikela, Mikele, Mikell, Mikella, Mikesha, Mikeya, Mikhaela, Mikie, Mikiela, Mikkel, Mikyla, Mykaela

Mildred (English) gentle counselor.
Mil, Mila, Mildrene, Mildrid, Millie, Milly

Millicent (Greek) an alternate form of Melissa. (English) industrious.

Millicent *(cont.)*
Melicent, Meliscent,
Melly, Milicent, Milisent,
Millie, Missy

Mina (German) love.
(Persian) blue sky. (Hindi)
born in the lunar month
of Pisces. (Arabic) harbor.
(Japanese) south. A short
form of names ending in
"mina."
Meena, Mena, Min

Mindy (Greek) a familiar
form of Melinda.
Mindee, Mindi, Mindie,
Mindyanne, Mindylee,
Myndy

Miranda (Latin) strange;
wonderful; admirable.
Literature: the heroine of
Shakespeare's *The Tempest.*
See also Randi.
Maranda, Marenda,
Meranda, Mira, Miran,
Miranada, Mirandia,
Mirinda, Mirindé,
Mironda, Mirranda,
Muranda, Myranda

Mireille (Hebrew) God
spoke. (Latin) wonderful.
Mirella, Mirelle, Mirelys,
Mireya, Mireyda, Mirielle,
Mirilla, Myrella, Myrilla

Miriam (Hebrew) bitter,
sea of bitterness. Bible:
the original form of Mary.
Marca, Marcsa, Mariam,
Mariame, Meryem,
Miram, Mirham, Miri,

Miriain, Miriama,
Miriame, Mirian, Mirit,
Mirjam, Mirjana, Mirra,
Mirriam, Mirrian, Miryam,
Miryan, Myriam

Missy (English) a familiar
form of Melissa, Millicent.
Missi, Missie

Misty (English) shrouded
by mist.
Missty, Mistee, Mistey,
Misti, Mistie, Mistin,
Mistina, Mistral,
Mistylynn, Mystee, Mysti,
Mystie

Moira (Irish) great. A form
of Mary. See also Maura.
Mayra, Moirae, Moirah,
Moire, Moya, Moyra,
Moyrah

Molly (Irish) a familiar form
of Mary.
Moll, Mollee, Molley,
Molli, Mollie, Mollissa

Mona (Greek) a short form
of Monica, Ramona. (Irish)
noble.
Moina, Monah, Mone,
Monea, Monna, Moyna

Monica (Greek) solitary.
(Latin) advisor.
Mona, Monca, Monee,
Monia, Monic, Monice,
Monicia, Monicka,
Monika, Monique,
Monise, Monn, Monnica,
Monnie, Monya

Monique (French) a form
of Monica.

Moniqua, Moniquea, Moniquie, Munique

Morgan (Welsh) seashore. Literature: Morgan Le Fay was the half-sister of King Arthur.
Morgana, Morgance, Morgane, Morganetta, Morganette, Morganica, Morgann, Morganna, Morganne, Morgen, Morgyn, Morrigan

Moriah (Hebrew) God is my teacher. (French) dark skinned. Bible: the name of the mountain on which the temple of Solomon was built. See also Mariah.
Moria, Moriel, Morit, Morria, Morriah

Muriel (Arabic) myrrh. (Irish) shining sea. A form of Mary. See also Meryl.
Murial, Muriell, Murielle

Mylene (Greek) dark.
Mylaine, Mylana, Mylee, Myleen, Mylenda, Mylinda

Myra (Latin) fragrant ointment. A feminine form of Myron.
Myrena, Myria

Myriam (American) a form of Miriam.
Myriame, Myryam

N

Nada (Arabic) generous; dewy.
Nadda

Nadia (French, Slavic) hopeful.
Nada, Nadea, Nadezhda, Nadie, Nadine, Nadiya, Nadja, Nady, Nadya

Nadine (French, Slavic) a form of Nadia.
Nadean, Nadeana, Nadeen, Nadena, Nadene, Nadien, Nadina, Nadyne, Naidene, Naidine

Nakia (Arabic) pure.
Nakea, Nakeia

Nakita (American) a form of Nicole, Nikita.
Nakia, Nakkita, Naquita

Nancy (English) gracious.
Nainsi, Nance, Nancee, Nancey, Nanci, Nancie, Nancine, Nancsi, Nancye, Nanette, Nanice, Nanine, Nanncey, Nanncy, Nanouk, Nansee, Nansey, Nanuk, Noni, Nonie

Naomi (Hebrew) pleasant, beautiful. Bible: a friend of Ruth.

Naomi (cont.)
Naoma, Naomia, Naomie, Naomy, Navit, Neoma, Neomi, Noami, Noemi, Noemie, Noma, Nomi, Nyome, Nyomi

Natalia (Russian) a form of Natalie.
Nacia, Natala, Nataliia, Natalina, Natalja, Natalya, Nathalia

Natalie (Latin) born on Christmas day. See also Natasha, Noel.
Nat, Natalea, Natalee, Natalene, Natalène, Natali, Natalia, Natalija, Nataline, Natalle, Nataly, Natalya, Natalyn, Natelie, Nathalia, Nathalie, Nathaly, Nati, Natie, Natilie, Natlie, Nattalie, Natti, Nattie, Nattilie, Nattlee, Natty

Natasha (Russian) a form of Natalie. See also Stacey, Tasha.
Nahtasha, Natacha, Natachia, Natacia, Natasa, Natascha, Natashah, Natashea, Natashia, Natashiea, Natashja, Natasia, Natassija, Natassja, Natasza, Natausha, Natawsha, Nathasha, Nathassha, Naticha, Natisha, Natishia, Natosha, Natoshia, Netasha, Netosha, Notasha, Notosha

Nellie (English) a familiar form of Eleanor, Helen.
Nel, Neli, Nell, Nella, Nelley, Nelli, Nellianne, Nellice, Nellis, Nelly, Nelma

Nia (Irish) a familiar form of Neila. Mythology: a legendary Welsh woman.
Niah, Nya, Nyah

Nichelle (American) a combination of Nicole + Michelle. Culture: Nichelle Nichols was the first African American woman featured in a television drama *Star Trek*.
Nichele, Nishelle

Nichole (French) an alternate form of Nicole.
Nichol, Nichola

Nicki (French) a familiar form of Nicole.
Nicci, Nickey, Nickeya, Nickia, Nickie, Nickiya, Nicky, Niki

Nicola (Italian) a form of Nicole.
Nacola, Necola, Nichola, Nickola, Nicolea, Nicolla, Nikkola, Nikola, Nikolia, Nykola

Nicole (French) victorious people. A feminine form of Nicholas. See also Colette, Nikita.
Nacole, Nakita, Necole, Nica, Nichol, Nichole, Nicholette, Nicia, Nicki,

**Nickol, Nickole, Nicol,
Nicola, Nicolette, Nicoli,
Nicolie, Nicoline, Nicolle,
Nikki, Niquole, Nocole**

Nicolette (French) an alternate form of Nicole.
**Nettie, Nicholette,
Nicoletta, Nikkolette,
Nikoleta, Nikoletta,
Nikolette**

Nicolle (French) an alternate form of Nicole.
Nicholle

Niesha (American) pure.
**Neisha, Neishia, Neissia,
Nesha, Neshia, Nesia,
Nessia, Niessia, Nisha**

Nika (Russian) belonging to God.

Niki (Russian) a short form of Nikita.
Nikia

Nikita (Russian) victorious people. A form of Nicole.
**Niki, Nikki, Nikkita,
Niquita, Niquitta**

Nikki (American) a familiar form of Nicole, Nikita.
**Nicki, Nikia, Nikka,
Nikkey, Nikkia, Nikkie,
Nikky**

Nikole (French) an alternate form of Nicole.
**Nikkole, Nikola, Nikole,
Nikolle**

Nina (Hebrew) a familiar form of Hannah. (Spanish) girl. (Native American) mighty.
**Neena, Nena, Ninacska,
Nineta, Ninete, Ninetta,
Ninette, Ninita, Ninja,
Ninnetta, Ninnette,
Ninon, Ninosca, Ninoshka,
Nynette**

Nisha (American) an alternate form of Niesha.

Nita (Hebrew) planter.
(Spanish) a short form of Anita, Juanita.
(Choctaw) bear.
Nitika

Noel (Latin) Christmas.
**Noël, Noela, Noeleen,
Noelene, Noelia, Noeline,
Noelle, Noelyn, Noelynn,
Noleen, Novelenn,
Novelia, Nowel, Noweleen,
Nowell**

Noelle (French) Christmas.
A form of Noel.
**Noell, Noella, Noelleen,
Noellyn**

Noemi (Hebrew) an alternate form of Naomi.
Noemie, Nohemi, Nomi

Nora (Greek) light.
A familiar form of Eleanor.
Norah, Noreen

Noreen (Irish) a form of Eleanor, Nora. (Latin) a familiar form of Norma.
**Noorin, Noreena, Noren,
Norene, Norina, Norine,
Nureen**

Norma (Latin) rule, precept.
Noma, Noreen, Normi, Normie

Nyssa (Greek) beginning.
Nisha, Nissi, Nissy, Nysa

O

Octavia (Latin) eighth.
See also Tavia.
Octavice, Octavie, Octavienne, Octavise, Octivia, Ottavia

Olga (Scandinavian) holy.
See also Olivia.
Olenka, Olia, Olva

Olivia (Latin) olive tree.
(English) a form of Olga.
Oliva, Olive, Olivea, Olivetta, Olivianne, Oliwia, Ollie, Olly, Ollye, Olva, Olyvia

Ondine (Latin) little wave.
Ondina, Ondyne

Oprah (Hebrew) runaway.
Ophra, Ophrah, Opra

P

Paige (English) young child.

Pamela (Greek) honey.
Pam, Pama, Pamala, Pamalla, Pamelia, Pamelina, Pamella, Pamilla, Pammela, Pammi, Pammie, Pammy, Pamula

Paola (Italian) a form of Paula.
Paolina

Paris (French) Geography: the capital of France.
Mythology: the Trojan prince who started the Trojan war by abducting Helen.
Parice, Paries, Parisa, Pariss, Parissa, Parris

Patience (English) patient.
Paciencia, Patia, Patty

Patrice (French) a form of Patricia.
Patrease, Patrece, Patresa, Patriece, Patryce, Pattrice

Patricia (Latin) noble-woman. A feminine form of Patrick. See also Tricia, Trisha.

**Pat, Patia, Patreece,
Patreice, Patrica, Patrice,
Patriceia, Patricja,
Patricka, Patrickia,
Patrisha, Patrishia,
Patrizia, Patrizzia, Patsy,
Patty**

Paula (Latin) small. A feminine form of Paul.
**Pali, Paliki, Paola,
Paulane, Paulann, Paule,
Paulette, Pauli, Paulie,
Pauline, Paulla, Pauly,
Pavia, Polly**

Paulette (Latin) a familiar form of Paula.
**Pauletta, Paulita,
Paullette**

Pauline (Latin) a familiar form of Paula.
**Pauleen, Paulene, Paulina,
Paulyne, Pawlina**

Pearl (Latin) jewel.
**Pearla, Pearle, Pearleen,
Pearlena, Pearlene,
Pearlette, Pearlie,
Pearline, Perlette, Perlie,
Perline, Perlline, Perry**

Peggy (Greek) a familiar form of Margaret.
**Peg, Pegeen, Pegg,
Peggey, Peggi, Peggie,
Pegi**

Penny (Greek) weaver.
**Penee, Penney, Penni,
Pennie**

Petra (Greek, Latin) small rock. A feminine form of Peter.

**Pet, Peta, Petena,
Peterina, Petrice, Petrina,
Petrine, Pier, Pierette,
Pierrette, Pietra**

Philippa (Greek) lover of horses. A feminine form of Philip.
**Phil, Philipa, Philippe,
Phillipina, Phillippine,
Phillie, Philly, Pippa,
Pippy**

Phoebe (Greek) shining.
**Phaebe, Pheba, Phebe,
Pheby, Phoebey**

Phylicia (Greek) a form of Felicia. (Latin) fortunate; happy.
**Philica, Philycia, Phylecia,
Phylesia, Phylisha,
Phylisia, Phyllecia,
Phyllicia, Phyllisia**

Phyllis (Greek) green bough.
**Filise, Fillys, Fyllis, Philis,
Phillis, Philliss, Philys,
Philyss, Phylis, Phyllida,
Phyllis, Phylliss, Phyllys**

Porsche (German) a form of Portia.
**Porcha, Porchai, Porcsha,
Porcshe, Porscha, Porsché,
Porschea, Porschia,
Pourche**

Porsha (Latin) an alternate form of Portia.
**Porshai, Porshay, Porshe,
Porshia**

Portia (Latin) offering. Literature: the heroine of Shakespeare's play *The Merchant of Venice*.
Porsche, Porsha, Portiea

Precious (French) precious; dear.

Princess (English) daughter of royalty.
Princcess, Princetta, Princie, Princilla

Priscilla (Latin) ancient.
Cilla, Piri, Precilla, Prescilla, Pricila, Pricilla, Pris, Prisca, Priscella, Priscila, Priscill, Priscille, Prisella, Prisila, Prisilla, Prissilla, Prissy, Prysilla

Priya (Hindi) beloved; sweet natured.

Q

Queisha (American) a combination of the prefix Qu + Aisha.
Qeysha, Queshia

Quiana (American) a combination of the prefix Qu + Anna.
Quian, Quianna

Quinn (German, English) queen. See also Queenie.
Quin, Quinna

Quintana (Latin) fifth. (English) queen's lawn. A feminine form of Quentin, Quintin.
Quinntina, Quinta, Quintanna, Quintara, Quintarah, Quintia, Quintila, Quintilla, Quintina, Quintona, Quintonice

R

Rachael (Hebrew) an alternate form of Rachel.
Rachaele

Rachel (Hebrew) female sheep. Bible: the wife of Jacob. See also Rae, Rochelle.
Racha, Rachael, Rachal, Racheal, Rachela, Rachelann, Rachele, Rachelle, Rackel, Raechel, Raechele, Rahel, Rahela, Rahil, Rakel, Rakhil, Raquel, Ray, Raycene, Rey, Ruchel

Rachelle (French) a form of Rachel. See also Shelley.
Rachalle, Rachell, Rachella, Raechell, Raechelle, Raeshelle, Rashel, Rashele, Rashell,

Rashelle, Raychell, Rayshell, Rochell, Ruchelle

Racquel (French) a form of Rachel.
Racquell, Racquella, Racquelle

Rae (English) doe. (Hebrew) a short form of Rachel.
Raeda, Raedeen, Raeden, Raeh, Raelene, Raena, Raenah, Raeneice, Raeneisha, Raesha, Raewyn, Ralina, Ray, Raye, Rayetta, Rayette, Rayma, Rayna, Rayona, Rey

Raeann (American) a combination of Rae + Ann.
Raea, Raeanna, Reanna, Raeanne

Raina (German) mighty. (English) a short form of Regina. See also Rayna.
Raenah, Raheena, Raine, Rainna, Reanna

Ramona (Spanish) mighty; wise protector. See also Mona.
Ramonda, Raymona, Romona, Romonda

Randall (English) protected.
Randa, Randah, Randal, Randalee, Randel, Randell, Randelle, Randi, Randilee, Randilynn, Randlyn, Randy, Randyl

Randi, Randy (English) familiar forms of Miranda, Randall.
Rande, Randee, Randeen, Randene, Randey, Randie, Randii

Raquel (French) a form of Rachel.
Rakel, Rakhil, Rakhila, Raqueal, Raquela, Raquella, Raquelle, Rickquel, Ricquel, Ricquelle, Rikell, Rikelle, Rockell

Rashida (Swahili, Turkish) righteous.
Rahshea, Rahsheda, Rahsheita, Rashdah, Rasheda, Rashedah, Rasheeda, Rasheeta, Rasheida, Rashidi

Raven (English) blackbird.
Raveen, Raveena, Ravena, Ravennah, Ravi, Ravin, Ravine, Ravyn, Rayven, Rayvin

Rayna (Scandinavian) mighty. (Yiddish) pure, clean. (French) a familiar form of Lorraine. (English) king's advisor. A feminine form of Reynold. See also Raina.
Rayna, Rayne, Raynell, Raynelle, Raynette, Rayona, Rayonna, Reyna

Reanna (German, English) an alternate form of Raina

Reanna *(cont.)*
(American) an alternate
form of Raeann.
Reannah

Reba (Hebrew) fourth-born
child. A short form of
Rebecca. See also Reva.
Rabah, Reeba, Rheba

Rebecca (Hebrew) tied,
bound. Bible: the wife
of Isaac. See also Becky.
**Becca, Rabecca, Rabecka,
Reba, Rebbecca, Rebeca,
Rebeccah, Rebeccea,
Rebeccka, Rebecha,
Rebecka, Rebeckah,
Rebeckia, Rebecky,
Rebekah, Rebeque, Rebi,
Reveca, Riva, Rivka**

Rebekah (Hebrew) an
alternate form of Rebecca.
**Rebeka, Rebekha,
Rebekka, Rebekkah,
Rebekke, Revecca, Reveka,
Revekka, Rifka**

Reena (Greek) peaceful.
Reen, Reenie, Rena, Reyna

Regan (Irish) little ruler.
Ragan, Reagan, Regin

Regina (Latin) queen.
(English) king's advisor.
A feminine form of
Reginald. Geography: the
capital of Saskatchewan.
See also Gina.
**Ragina, Raina, Raine,
Rane, Rega, Regena,
Regennia, Reggi, Reggie,
Reggy, Regi, Regia, Regie,**

**Regiena, Regin, Regine,
Reginia, Regis, Reina,
Rena**

Reina (Spanish) a short
form of Regina. See also
Reyna.
**Reine, Reinette, Reiny,
Reiona, Renia, Rina**

Rena (Hebrew) song; joy.
A familiar form of Irene,
Regina, Renata, Sabrina,
Serena.
**Reena, Rina, Rinna,
Rinnah**

Renae (French) an alternate
form of Renee.
Renay

Renata (French) an alter-
nate form of Renee.
**Ranata, Rena, Renada,
Renita, Rennie, Renyatta,
Rinada, Rinata**

Rene (Greek) a short form
of Irene, Renee.
**Reen, Reenie, Renae,
Reney, Rennie**

Renee (French) born again.
**Renae, Renata, Renay,
Rene, Renée, Renell,
Renelle**

Renita (French) an alternate form of Renata.
Reneeta, Renetta, Renitza

Reva (Latin) revived.
(Hebrew) rain; one-
fourth. An alternate
form of Reba.
Ree, Reeva, Revia, Revida

Reyna (Greek) peaceful. (English) an alternate form of Reina.
Reyne

Rhea (Greek) brook, stream. Mythology: the mother of Zeus.
Rheá, Rhéa, Rhealyn, Rheana, Rheann, Rheanna, Rheannan, Rheanne, Rheannon

Rhiannon (Welsh) witch; nymph; goddess.
Rhian, Rhiana, Rhianen, Rhianna, Rhianne, Rhiannen, Rhianon, Rhianwen, Rhiauna, Rhinnon, Rhyan, Rhyanna, Rian, Riana, Riane, Riann, Rianna, Rianne, Riannon, Rianon, Riayn

Rhoda (Greek) from Rhodes.
Rhode, Rhodeia, Rhodie, Rhody, Roda, Rodi, Rodie, Rodina

Rhonda (Welsh) grand.
Rhondelle, Rhondene, Rhondiesha, Rhonnie, Ronda, Ronelle, Ronnette

Richelle (German, French) rich and powerful ruler. A feminine form of Richard.
Richel, Richela, Richele, Richell, Richella, Richia

Ricki, Rikki (American) familiar forms of Erica.
Rica, Rici, Ricka, Rickia, Rickie, Rickilee, Rickina, Rickita, Ricky, Ricquie, Riki, Rikia, Rikita, Rikky

Riley (Irish) valiant.
Rileigh, Rilie

Rita (Sanskrit) brave; honest. (Greek) a short form of Margarita.
Reatha, Reda, Reeta, Reida, Reitha, Rheta, Riet, Ritamae, Ritamarie

Roberta (English) famous brilliance. A feminine form of Robert. See also Bobbi, Robin.
Roba, Robbi, Robbie, Robby, Robena, Robertena, Robertina

Robin (English) robin. An alternate form of Roberta.
Robann, Robbi, Robbie, Robbin, Robby, Robena, Robina, Robine, Robinette, Robinia, Robinn, Robinta, Robyn

Robyn (English) an alternate form of Robin.
Robbyn, Robyne, Robynn, Robynne

Rochelle (Hebrew) an alternate form of Rachel. (French) large stone. See also Shelley.
Roch, Rochele, Rochell, Rochella, Rochette, Rockelle, Roshele, Roshell, Roshelle

Rocio (Spanish) dewdrops.
Rocío

Ronda (Welsh) an alternate
form of Rhonda.
**Rondai, Rondel, Rondelle,
Rondesia, Rondi, Ronelle,
Ronndelle, Ronnette,
Ronni, Ronnie, Ronny**

Rosa (Italian, Spanish)
a form of Rose. History:
Rosa Parks inspired the
American civil rights
movement by refusing
to give up her bus seat
to a white man in
Montgomery, Alabama.
Roza

Rosalie (English) a form
of Rosalind.
**Rosalea, Rosalee,
Rosaleen, Rosalene,
Rosalia, Roselia, Rosilee,
Rosli, Rozali, Rozalie,
Rozália, Rozele**

Rosalind (Spanish) fair
rose.
**Ros, Rosalina, Rosalinda,
Rosalinde, Rosalyn,
Rosalynd, Rosalynde,
Roselind, Rosie, Rozalind**

Rosalyn (Spanish) an alter-
nate form of Rosalind.
**Ros, Rosaleen, Rosalin,
Rosaline, Rosalyne,
Rosalynn, Rosalynne,
Roseleen, Roselin,
Roseline, Roselyn,
Roselynn, Roselynne,
Rosilyn, Roslin, Roslyn,
Roslyne, Roslynn, Rozalyn,
Rozland, Rozlyn**

Rosanna, Roseanna
(English) combinations
of Rose + Anna.
**Ranna, Roanna, Rosana,
Rosannah, Roseana,
Roseannah, Rosehanah,
Rosehannah, Rosie,
Rossana, Rossanna,
Rozana, Rozanna**

Rosanne, Roseanne
(English) combinations
of Rose + Anne.
**Roanne, Rosan, Rosann,
Roseann, Rose Ann, Rose
Anne, Rossann, Rossanne,
Rozann, Rozanne**

Rose (Latin) rose.
**Rada, Rasia, Rasine, Rois,
Róise, Rosa, Rosella,
Roselle, Roseta, Rosetta,
Rosette, Rosie, Rosina,
Rosita, Rosse**

Rosemarie (English)
a combination of
Rose + Marie.
**Romy, Rosemaria, Rose
Marie**

Rosemary (English) a combination of Rose + Mary.
Romi, Romy

Rosetta (Italian) a form
of Rose.

Roxana, Roxanna
(Persian) alternate forms
of Roxann, Roxanne.
Rocsana

Roxann, Roxanne
(Persian) sunrise.
Literature: the heroine
of Edmond Rostand's play
Cyrano de Bergerac.
**Rocxann, Roxana, Roxane,
Roxanna, Roxianne, Roxy**

Ruby (French) precious
stone.
**Rubetta, Rubette, Rubey,
Rubi, Rubia, Rubiann,
Rubie, Rubyann, Rubye**

Ruth (Hebrew) friendship.
Bible: friend of Naomi.
**Rutha, Ruthalma, Ruthe,
Ruthella, Ruthetta, Ruthi,
Ruthie, Ruthina, Ruthine,
Ruthven, Ruthy**

Ryan (Irish) little ruler.
**Raiann, Raianne, Rhyann,
Riana, Riane, Ryana,
Ryann, Ryanna, Ryanne,
Rye, Ryen, Ryenne**

S

Sabina (Latin) History:
the Sabine were a tribe in
ancient Italy.
**Bina, Sabienne, Sabine,
Sabinka, Sabinna, Sabiny,
Saby, Sabyne, Savina,
Sebina, Sebinah**

Sable (English) sable; sleek.
Sabel, Sabela, Sabella

Sabra (Hebrew) thorny
cactus fruit. History:
a name for native-born
Israelis, who were said
to be hard on the outside
and soft and sweet on the
inside. (Arabic) resting.
**Sabira, Sabrah, Sabriya,
Sebra**

Sabrina (Latin) boundary
line. (Hebrew) a familiar
form of Sabra. (English)
princess. See also Bree,
Rena.
**Brina, Sabre, Sabreena,
Sabrinia, Sabrinna,
Sabryna, Sebree, Sebrina**

Sacha (Russian) an alternate form of Sasha.

Sade (Hebrew) an alternate
form of Sarah, Shardae.
Sáde, Sadé, Sadee

Sadie (Hebrew) a familiar
form of Sarah.
**Sadah, Sadella, Sadelle,
Sady, Sadye, Saidee,
Saydie, Sydel, Sydell,
Sydella, Sydelle**

Safiya (Arabic) pure;
serene; best friend.
**Safa, Safeya, Saffa, Safia,
Safiyah**

Salena (French) solemn,
dignified.
Saleena, Salina, Salinda

Sally (English) princess.
A familiar form of Sarah.
History: Sally Ride,
an American astronaut,
became the first U.S.
woman in space.
**Sal, Salaid, Sallee,
Salletta, Sallette, Salley,
Salli, Salliann, Sallie**

Samantha (Aramaic)
listener. (Hebrew) told
by God.
**Sam, Samana, Samanath,
Samanatha, Samanitha,
Samanithia, Samanta,
Samanth, Samanthe,
Samanthi, Samanthia,
Sami, Sammanth,
Sammantha, Sammatha,
Semantha, Simantha,
Smanta, Smantha,
Symantha**

Samara (Latin) elm tree
seed.
**Sam, Samaria, Samarie,
Samarra, Samera,
Sameria, Samira, Sammar,
Sammara, Samora**

Sana (Arabic) mountaintop;
splendid; brilliant.
Sanaa, Sanáa

Sandeep (Punjabi)
enlightened.

Sandi (Greek) a familiar
form of Sandra.
**Sandee, Sandia, Sandie,
Sandiey, Sandine, Sanndie**

Sandra (Greek) defender
of mankind. A short form
of Alexandra, Cassandra.
History: Sandra Day
O'Connor was the first
woman appointed to the
U.S. Supreme Court.
**Sahndra, Sandi, Sandira,
Sandrea, Sandria,
Sandrica, Sandy, Saundra,
Shandra, Sondra, Zandra**

Sandy (Greek) a familiar
form of Cassandra, Sandra.
Sandya, Sandye

Santana (Spanish) saint.
**Santa, Santaniata,
Santanna, Santanne,
Santena, Santenna,
Santina, Shantana**

Sara (Hebrew) an alternate
form of Sarah.
Saralee, Sarra

Sarah (Hebrew) princess.
Bible: the wife of Abraham
and mother of Isaac.
See also Sadie, Sally, Sari,
Sharaya, Shari, Zara.
**Sahra, Sara, Saraha,
Sarahann, Sarai, Sarann,
Sarina, Sarita, Sarolta,
Sarotte, Sarrah, Sasa,
Sayre, Sorcha**

Sari (Hebrew) a familiar
form of Sarah. (Arabic)
noble.
**Saree, Sareeka, Sareka,
Sarika, Sarka, Sarri,
Sarrie, Sary**

Sarina (Hebrew) a familiar
form of Sarah.

**Sareen, Sarena, Sarene,
Sarinna, Sarinne**

Sarita (Hebrew) a familiar
form of Sarah.
**Saretta, Sarette, Saritia,
Sarolta, Sarotte**

Sasha (Russian) defender
of mankind. A short form
of Alexandra.
**Sacha, Sahsha,
Sasa, Sascha, Saschae,
Sashah, Sashana, Sashel,
Sashia, Sashira, Sashsha,
Sasjara, Sasshalai, Sausha,
Shasha, Shashi, Shashia,
Shura**

Saundra (English) a form
of Sandra, Sondra.
**Saundee, Saundi, Saundie,
Saundy**

Savannah (Spanish) tree-
less plain.
**Sahvannah, Savana,
Savanah, Savanha,
Savanna, Savannha,
Savauna, Sevan, Sevanah,
Sevanh, Sevann, Sevanna,
Svannah**

Scarlett (English) bright
red. Literature: Scarlett
O'Hara is the heroine
of Margaret Mitchell's
novel *Gone with the Wind*.
**Scarlet, Scarlette,
Scarlotte, Skarlette**

Selena (Greek) moon.
Mythology: Selene was
the goddess of the moon.
See also Celena.

**Saleena, Sela, Selen,
Selene, Séléné, Selenia,
Selina, Sena, Syleena,
Sylena**

Selina (Greek) an alternate
form of Celina, Selena.
**Selia, Selie, Selina,
Selinda, Seline, Selinka,
Selyna, Selyne, Sylina**

Serena (Latin) peaceful.
See also Rena.
**Sarina, Saryna, Sereena,
Serenah, Serene, Serenity,
Serenna, Serina, Serrena,
Serrin, Serrina, Seryna**

Shae (Irish) an alternate
form of Shea.
**Shaeen, Shaeine, Shaela,
Shaelea, Shaelee,
Shaeleigh, Shaelie, Shaely,
Shaelyn, Shaena, Shaenel,
Shaeya, Shaia**

Shaina (Yiddish) beautiful.
**Shaena, Shainah, Shaine,
Shainna, Shajna, Shanie,
Shayna, Shayndel, Sheina,
Sheindel**

Shakia (American)
a combination of the
prefix Sha + Kia.
**Shakeeia, Shakeeyah,
Shakeia, Shakeya,
Shakiya, Shekeia, Shekia,
Shekiah, Shikia**

Shakira (Arabic) thankful.
A feminine form of Shakir.
**Shaakira, Shaka, Shakera,
Shakerah, Shakeria,
Shakeriay, Shakeyra,**

Shakira *(cont.)*
Shakir, Shakirah,
Shakirat, Shakirra,
Shakyra, Shekiera,
Shekira, Shikira

Shakita (American)
a combination of the
prefix Sha + Kita.
See also Shaquita.
Shaka, Shakeeta,
Shaketa, Shaketha,
Shakethia, Shaketia,
Sheketa, Shekita

Shalana (American)
a combination of the
prefix Sha + Lana.
Shalaina, Shalaine,
Shalane, Shalann

Shalonda (American)
a combination of the
prefix Sha + Ondine.
Shalonde, Shalondine

Shameka (American)
a combination of the
prefix Sha + Meka.
Shameca, Shamecca,
Shamecha, Shameeka,
Shameika, Shameke,
Shamekia

Shamika (American)
a combination of the
prefix Sha + Mika.
Shamica, Shamicia,
Shamicka, Shamieka,
Shamikia

Shamira (Hebrew) precious
stone.
Shamir, Shamiran,
Shamiria

Shana (Hebrew) God is
gracious. (Irish) a form
of Jane.
Shaana, Shan, Shanae,
Shanay, Shanda, Shandi,
Shane, Shanna, Shannah,
Shauna, Shawna

Shanae (Irish) an alternate
form of Shana.
Shanea

Shanda (American) a form
of Chanda, Shana.
Shandah

Shandi (English) a familiar
form of Shana.
Shandee, Shandeigh,
Shandey, Shandi,
Shandice, Shandie

Shandra (American) an
alternate form of Shanda.
See also Chandra.
Shandrea, Shandreka,
Shandri, Shandria,
Shandriah, Shandrice,
Shandrie, Shandry

Shaneka (American)
an alternate form of
Shanika.
Shanecka, Shaneikah,
Shanekia, Shanequa,
Shaneyka

Shanel, Shanell, Shanelle
(American) forms
of Chanel.
Schanel, Schanell,
Shanella, Shannel, Shenel,
Shenela, Shenell, Shenelle,
Shonelle, Shynelle

Shani (Swahili) marvelous.

Shanika (American)
a combination of the
prefix Sha + Nika.
**Shanica, Shanicca,
Shanicka, Shanieka,
Shanike, Shanikia,
Shanikka, Shanikqua,
Shanikwa, Shaniqua,
Shanique, Shenika**

Shanita (American)
a combination of the
prefix Sha + Nita.
**Shanitha, Shanitra,
Shanitta**

Shanna (Irish) an alternate
form of Shana, Shannon.
**Shanea, Shannah,
Shannda, Shannea**

Shannon (Irish) small and
wise.
**Shanan, Shann, Shanna,
Shannan, Shanneen,
Shannen, Shannie,
Shannin, Shannyn,
Shanon**

Shanta, Shantae, Shante
(French) alternate forms
of Chantal.
**Shantai, Shantay,
Shantaya, Shantaye,
Shantea, Shantee,
Shantée**

Shantel, Shantell
(American) song.
Forms of Chantel.
**Shanntell, Shanta,
Shantal, Shantae,
Shantale, Shante,**

**Shanteal, Shanteil,
Shantele, Shantella,
Shantelle, Shantrell,
Shantyl, Shantyle,
Shauntel, Shauntell,
Shauntelle, Shauntrel,
Shauntrell, Shauntrella,
Shentel, Shentelle,
Shontal, Shontalla,
Shontalle**

Shaquita (American)
an alternate form
of Shakita.
Shaqueta, Shaquetta

Shara (Hebrew) a short
form of Sharon.
**Shaara, Sharal, Sharala,
Sharalee, Sharlyn,
Sharlynn, Sharra**

Sharaya (Hebrew) princess.
An alternate form of Sarah.
See also Sharon.
**Sharae, Sharaé, Sharah,
Sharai, Sharaiah, Sharay**

Shardae, Sharday
(Punjabi) charity. (Yoruba)
honored by royalty.
(Arabic) runaway. An alter-
nate form of Chardae.
**Sade, Shadae, Sharda,
Shar-Dae, Shardai, Shar-
Day, Sharde, Shardea,
Shardee, Shardée,
Shardei, Shardeia,
Shardey**

Sharee (English) a form
of Shari.
**Shareen, Shareena,
Sharine**

Shari (French) beloved,
dearest. An alternate form
of Cheri. (Hungarian) a
form of Sarah. See also
Sharita, Sheree, Sherry.
**Shara, Sharee, Sharian,
Shariann, Sharianne,
Sharie, Sharra, Sharree,
Sharrie, Sharry, Shary**

Sharita (French) a familiar
form of Shari. (American)
a form of Charity. See also
Sherita.
Shareeta, Sharrita

Sharla (French) a short
form of Sharlene.

Sharlene (French) little
and womanly. A form
of Charlene.
**Scharlane, Scharlene,
Shar, Sharla, Sharlaina,
Sharlaine, Sharlane,
Sharlanna, Sharlee,
Sharleen, Sharleine,
Sharlena, Sharleyne,
Sharline, Sharlyn,
Sharlynn, Sharlynne,
Sherlean, Sherleen,
Sherlene, Sherline**

Sharon (Hebrew) desert
plain. An alternate form
of Sharaya.
**Shaaron, Shara, Sharai,
Sharan, Shareen, Sharen,
Shari, Sharin, Sharna,
Sharonda, Sharran,
Sharren, Sharrin, Sharron,
Sharrona, Sharyn,
Sharyon, Sheren, Sheron,
Sherryn**

Shatara (Hindi) umbrella.
(Arabic) good; industrious.
(American) a combination
of Sharon + Tara.
**Shataria, Shatarra,
Shataura, Shateira,
Shaterah, Shateria,
Shatherian, Shatierra,
Shatiria**

Shauna (Hebrew) God is
gracious. (Irish) an alter-
nate form of Shana.
**Shaun, Shaunah, Shaune,
Shaunee, Shauneen,
Shaunelle, Shaunette,
Shauni, Shaunice,
Shaunicy, Shaunie,
Shaunika, Shaunisha,
Shaunna, Shaunnea,
Shaunua, Shaunya**

Shaunda (Irish) an alter-
nate form of Shauna.
See also Shanda,
Shawnda, Shonda.
**Shaundal, Shaundala,
Shaundel, Shaundela,
Shaundell, Shaundelle,
Shaundra, Shaundrea,
Shaundree, Shaundria,
Shaundrice**

Shavonne (American)
a combination of the
prefix Sha + Yvonne.
See also Siobhan.
**Schavon, Schevon,
Shavan, Shavana,
Shavanna, Shavaun,
Shavon, Shavonda,
Shavondra, Shavone,
Shavonn, Shavonna,**

Shavonni, Shavontae,
Shavonte, Shavonté,
Shavoun, Shivani,
Shivaun, Shivawn,
Shivonne, Shyvon,
Shyvonne

Shawna (Hebrew) God is
gracious. (Irish) a form
of Jane. An alternate form
of Shana, Shauna.
Shawn, Shawnai, Shawne,
Shawnee, Shawneen,
Shawneena, Shawneika,
Shawnell, Shawnette,
Shawni, Shawnicka,
Shawnie, Shawnika,
Shawnna, Shawnra,
Sheona, Siân, Siana,
Sianna

Shawnda (Irish) an alter-
nate form of Shawna.
See also Shanda,
Shaunda, Shonda.
Shawndal, Shawndala,
Shawndan, Shawndel,
Shawndra, Shawndrea,
Shawndree, Shawndreel,
Shawndrell, Shawndria

Shay (Irish) an alternate
form of Shea.
Shaya, Shayda, Shaye,
Shayha, Shayia, Shey,
Sheye

Shayla (Irish) an alternate
form of Shay.
Shay, Shaylagh, Shaylah,
Shaylain, Shaylan,
Shaylea, Shaylee, Shayley,
Shayli, Shaylie, Shaylin,
Shaylla, Shayly, Shaylyn,
Shaylynn, Sheyla, Sheylyn

Shayna (Hebrew) beautiful.
A form of Shaina.
Shaynae, Shayne,
Shaynee, Shayney, Shayni,
Shaynie, Shayny

Shea (Irish) fairy palace.
Shae, Shay, Shealy,
Shealyn, Sheana, Sheann,
Sheanna, Sheannon,
Sheanta, Sheaon, Shearra,
Sheatara, Sheaunna,
Sheavon

Sheena (Hebrew) God is
gracious. (Irish) a form
of Jane.
Sheenagh, Sheenah,
Sheenan, Sheeneal,
Sheenika, Sheenna,
Sheina, Shena, Shiona

Sheila (Latin) blind. (Irish)
a form of Cecelia.
Seelia, Seila, Selia,
Shaylah, Sheela, Sheelagh,
Sheelah, Sheilagh,
Sheilah, Sheileen,
Sheiletta, Sheilia,
Sheillynn, Sheilya, Shela,
Shelagh, Shelah, Shelia,
Shiela, Shila, Shilah,
Shilea, Shyla

Shelby (English) ledge
estate.
Schelby, Shel, Shelbe,
Shelbee, Shelbey, Shelbi,
Shelbie, Shellby

Shelley, Shelly (English)
meadow on the ledge.

Shelley, Shelly *(cont.)*
(French) a familiar form
of Michelle. See also
Rachelle, Rochelle.
**Shelee, Shell, Shella,
Shellaine, Shellana,
Shellany, Shellee,
Shellene, Shelli, Shellian,
Shellie, Shellina**

Shena (Irish) an alternate
form of Sheena.
**Shenada, Shenae, Shenay,
Shenda, Shene, Shenea,
Sheneda, Shenee,
Sheneena, Shenica,
Shenika, Shenina,
Sheniqua, Shenita,
Shenna**

Shera (Aramaic) light.
**Sheera, Sheerah, Sherae,
Sherah, Sheralee, Sheralle,
Sheralyn, Sheralynn,
Sheralynne, Sheray,
Sheraya**

Sheree (French) beloved,
dearest. An alternate form
of Shari.
**Scherie, Sheeree, Shere,
Shereé, Sherrelle,
Shereen, Shereena**

Sherell (French) an alter-
nate form of Cherelle,
Sheryl.
Sherrell

Sheri, Sherri (French)
alternate forms of Sherry.
**Sheria, Sheriah, Sherian,
Sherianne, Shericia,**

**Sherie, Sheriel, Sherrie,
Sherrina**

Sherika (Punjabi) relative
(Arabic) easterner.
**Shereka, Sherica,
Shericka, Sherrica,
Sherricka, Sherrika**

Sherita (French) a form
of Sherry, Sheryl. See also
Sharita.
**Shereta, Sheretta,
Sherette, Sherrita**

Sherry (French) beloved,
dearest. An alternate form
of Shari. A familiar form
of Sheryl. See also Sheree.
**Sherey, Sheri, Sherissa,
Sherrey, Sherri, Sherria,
Sherriah, Sherrie, Sherye,
Sheryy**

Sheryl (French) beloved.
An alternate form of
Cheryl. A familiar form
of Shirley. See also Sherry.
**Sharel, Sharil, Sharilyn,
Sharyl, Sharyll, Sheral,
Sherell, Sheriel, Sheril,
Sherill, Sherily, Sherilyn,
Sherissa, Sherita,
Sherleen, Sherral, Sherrel,
Sherrell, Sherrelle, Sherril,
Sherrill, Sherryl, Sherylly**

Shilo (Hebrew) God's gift.
Geography: a site near
Jerusalem. Bible: a sanctu-
ary for the Israelites where
the Ark of the Covenant
was kept.
Shiloh

Shira (Hebrew) song.
Shirah, Shiray, Shire,
Shiree, Shiri, Shirit

Shirley (English) bright
meadow. See also Sheryl.
Sherlee, Sherleen, Sherley,
Sherli, Sherlie, Shir,
Shirelle, Shirl, Shirlee,
Shirlena, Shirlene, Shirlie,
Shirlina, Shirly, Shirlyn,
Shirlly, Shurlee, Shurley

Shona (Irish) a form of
Jane. An alternate form of
Shana, Shauna, Shawna.
Shonagh, Shonah,
Shonalee, Shonda,
Shone, Shonee, Shonelle,
Shonetta, Shonette,
Shoni, Shonna, Shonneka,
Shonnika, Shonta

Shonda (Irish) an alternate
form of Shona. See also
Shanda, Shaunda,
Shawnda.
Shondalette, Shondalyn,
Shondel, Shondelle,
Shondi, Shondia, Shondie,
Shondra, Shondreka,
Shounda

Shoshana (Hebrew) lily.
An alternate form of
Susan.
Shosha, Shoshan,
Shoshanah, Shoshane,
Shoshanha, Shoshann,
Shoshanna, Shoshannah,
Shoshauna, Shoushan,
Sosha, Soshana

Shyla (English) an alternate
form of Sheila.

Sierra (Irish) black.
(Spanish) saw toothed.
Geography: a rugged
range of mountains
that, when viewed from
a distance, has a jagged
profile. See also Ciara.
Seara, Searria, Seera,
Seiarra, Seira, Seirra,
Siara, Siarah, Siarra,
Sieara, Siearra, Siera,
Sieria, Sierrah, Sierre

Silvia (Latin) an alternate
form of Sylvia.
Silivia, Silva, Silvaine,
Silvanna, Silvi, Silviane,
Silva, Silvy

Simone (Hebrew) she
heard. (French) a feminine
form of Simon.
Siminie, Simmi, Simmie,
Simmona, Simmone,
Simoane, Simona,
Simonetta, Simonette,
Simonia, Simonina,
Simonne, Somone,
Symona, Symone

Siobhan (Irish) a form of
Joan. See also Shavonne.
Shibahn, Shibani,
Shibhan, Shioban,
Shobana, Shobha,
Shobhana, Siobahn,
Siobhana, Siobhann,
Siobhon, Siovaun, Siovhan

Skye (Arabic) water giver.
(Dutch) a short form
of Skyler. Geography:
an island in the Hebrides,
Scotland.
Sky

Sofia (Greek) an alternate
form of Sophia.
**Sofeea, Sofeeia, Soffi,
Sofi, Soficita, Sofie, Sofija,
Sofiya, Sofya, Zofia**

Sommer (English) summer;
summoner. (Arabic) black.
See also Summer.
Sommar, Sommara

Sondra (Greek) defender
of mankind. A short form
of Alexandra.
**Saundra, Sondre,
Sonndra, Sonndre**

Sonia (Russian, Slavic) an
alternate form of Sonya.
**Sonica, Sonida, Sonita,
Sonni, Sonnie, Sonny**

Sonja (Scandinavian)
a form of Sonya.
Sonjae, Sonjia

Sonya (Greek) wise.
(Russian, Slavic) a form
of Sophia.
Sonia, Sonja, Sunya

Sophia (Greek) wise.
See also Sonya.
Sofia, Sophie

Sophie (Greek) a familiar
form of Sophia.
Sophey, Sophi, Sophy

Stacey, Stacy (Greek)
resurrection. (Irish) a short
form of Anastasia,
Natasha.
**Stace, Stacee, Staceyan,
Staceyann, Staicy, Stasya,
Stayce, Staycee, Staci**

Staci (Greek) an alternate
form of Stacey.
**Stacci, Stacia, Stacie,
Stayci**

Stacia (English) a short
form of Anastasia.
Stasia, Staysha

Starr (English) star.
**Star, Staria, Starla, Starle,
Starlee, Starleen, Starlet,
Starlette, Starley,
Starlight, Starly, Starri,
Starria, Starrika, Starrsha,
Starsha, Starshanna**

Stefanie (Greek) an alter-
nate form of Stephanie.
**Stafani, Stafanie,
Staffany, Stefaney,
Stefani, Stefania,
Stefanié, Stefanija,
Stefannie, Stefany,
Stefcia, Stefenie, Steffane,
Steffani, Steffanie,
Steffany, Steffi, Stefka**

Stella (Latin) star. (French)
a familiar form of Estelle.
Steile, Stellina

Stephanie (Greek)
crowned. A feminine form
of Stephan. See also Stevie.
**Stamatios, Stefanie,
Steffie, Stepania,**

**Stephaija, Stephaine,
Stephana, Stephanas,
Stephane, Stephanee,
Stephaney, Stephani,
Stephania, Stephanida,
Stéphanie, Stephanine,
Stephann, Stephannie,
Stephany, Stephene,
Stephenie, Stephianie,
Stephney, Stesha,
Stevanee**

Stephenie (Greek) an alternate form of Stephanie.
Stephena

Stevie (Greek) a familiar form of Stephanie.
**Steva, Stevana, Stevanee,
Stevee, Stevena, Stevey,
Stevi, Stevy, Stevye**

Stormy (English) impetuous by nature.
**Storm, Storme, Stormi,
Stormie**

Sue (Hebrew) a short form of Susan, Susanna.
**Suann, Suanna, Suanne,
Sueanne, Suetta**

Summer (English) summertime. See also Sommer.
**Sumer, Summar,
Summerbreeze,
Summerhaze, Summerlee**

Sunny (English) bright, cheerful.
Sunni, Sunnie

Sunshine (English) sunshine.

Susan (Hebrew) lily.
See also Shoshana.

**Sawsan, Siusan, Sosana,
Sosanna, Sue, Suesan,
Sueva, Suisan, Suke,
Susann, Susanna, Susanne,
Suse, Susen, Susette,
Suson, Sussi, Suzan,
Suzane, Suzette, Suzzane**

Susanna, Susannah
(Hebrew) alternate forms of Susan.
**Sonel, Sue, Suesanna,
Susana, Susanah, Susie,
Suzana, Suzanna, Suzanne**

Susie (American) a familiar form of Susan, Susanna.
**Suse, Susey, Susi, Sussy,
Susy, Suze, Suzi, Suzie,
Suzy**

Suzanne (English) a form of Susan.
**Susanne, Suszanne,
Suzane, Suzann, Suzzann,
Suzzanne**

Suzette (French) a form of Susan.
Susetta, Susette, Suzetta

Sybil (Greek) prophet.
Mythology: sibyls were oracles who relayed the messages of the gods.
**Sebila, Sib, Sibbel,
Sibbella, Sibbie, Sibbill,
Sibby, Sibeal, Sibel, Sibilla,
Sibyl, Sibylla, Sibylle,
Sibylline, Sybella, Sybila,
Sybilla, Sybille, Syble**

Sydney (French) from Saint Denis, France.
A feminine form of Sidney

Sydney *(cont.)*
Sy, Syd, Sydania, Sydel,
Sydelle, Sydna, Sydnee,
Sydni, Sydnie, Sydny,
Sydnye, Syndona,
Syndonah, Syndonia

Sylvana (Latin) forest.
Sylva, Sylvaine, Sylvanna,
Sylvi, Sylvie, Sylvina,
Sylvinnia, Sylvonna

Sylvia (Latin) forest.
Literature: Sylvia Plath was
a well-known American
writer and poet. See also
Silvia.
Sylvana, Sylvette, Sylvie,
Sylwia

Syreeta (Hindi) good
traditions. (Arabic)
companion.

T

Tabatha (Greek, Aramaic)
an alternate form of
Tabitha.
Tabathe, Tabathia,
Tabbatha

Tabitha (Greek, Aramaic)
gazelle.
Tabatha, Tabbee,
Tabbetha, Tabbey, Tabbi,
Tabbie, Tabbitha, Tabby,
Tabetha, Tabithia,
Tabotha, Tabtha, Tabytha

Takia (Arabic) worshiper.
Takeiyah, Takeya, Takija,
Takiya, Takiyah, Takkia,
Taqiyya, Taquaia,
Taquaya, Taquiia, Tekeyia,
Tekiya, Tikia, Tykeia,
Tykia

Talia (Greek) blooming.
(Hebrew) dew from
heaven. (Latin, French)
birthday.
Tahlia, Tali, Taliah,
Taliatha, Talieya, Taliya,
Talley, Tallia, Tallie, Tally,
Tallya, Talya, Talyah, Tylia

Tamar (Hebrew) a short
form of Tamara. (Russian)
History: a twelfth-century
Georgian queen.
Tamer, Tamor, Tamour

Tamara (Hebrew) palm
tree. See also Tammy.
Tamar, Tamará, Tamarah,
Tamaria, Tamarin,
Tamarla, Tamarra,
Tamarria, Tamarrian,
Tamarsha, Tamary,
Tamer, Tamera, Tamerai,
Tameria, Tameriás,
Tamma, Tammara,
Tammera, Tamora,
Tamoya, Tamra, Tamura,
Tamyra, Temara,
Temarian, Thama,
Thamar, Thamara,
Thamarra, Thamer,
Timara, Timera, Tomara,
Tymara

Tameka (Aramaic) twin.
Tameca, Tamecia,
Tamecka, Tameeka,
Tamekia, Tamiecka,
Tamieka, Temeka,
Timeeka, Timeka,
Tomeka, Tomekia,
Trameika, Tymeka,
Tymmeeka, Tymmeka

Tamika (Japanese) child
of the people.
Tami, Tamica, Tamieka,
Tamike, Tamikia,
Tamikka, Tamiko,
Tamiqua, Tamiyo, Timika,
Timikia, Tomika, Tymika,
Tymmicka

Tamila (American)
a combination of the
prefix Ta + Mila.
Tamala, Tamela, Tamelia,
Tamilla, Tamille, Tamillia,
Tamilya

Tammi, Tammie (English)
alternate forms of Tammy.
Tami, Tamia, Tamiah,
Tamie, Tamijo, Tamiya

Tammy (Hebrew) a familiar
form of Tamara. (English)
twin.
Tamilyn, Tamlyn,
Tammee, Tammey,
Tammi, Tammie, Tamy,
Tamya

Tamra (Hebrew) a short
form of Tamara.
Tammra, Tamrah

Tana (Slavic) a short form
of Tanya.

Taina, Tanae, Tanaeah,
Tanah, Tanairi, Tanairy,
Tanalia, Tanara, Tanas,
Tanasha, Tanashea,
Tanavia, Tanaya, Tanaz,
Tanea, Tania, Tanna,
Tannah

Taneisha, Tanesha
(American) a combination
of the prefix Ta + Niesha.
Tahniesha, Tanasha,
Tanashia, Taneesha,
Taneshea, Taneshia,
Tanesia, Tanesian,
Tanessa, Tanessia,
Taniesha, Tanneshia,
Tanniecia, Tanniesha,
Tantashea

Tania (Russian, Slavic) fairy
queen. A form of Tanya.
Taneea, Tanija, Tanika,
Tanis, Taniya, Tannia,
Tannica, Tannis, Tanniya,
Tannya, Tarnia

Tanis, Tannis (Slavic)
forms of Tania, Tanya.
Tanesa, Tanese, Taniese,
Tanisa, Tanissa, Tanka,
Tannesa, Tannese,
Tanniece, Tanniese,
Tannisa, Tannise, Tannus,
Tannyce, Tenice, Tenise,
Tennessa, Tonise, Tranice,
Tranise, Tranissa, Tynice,
Tyniece, Tyniese, Tynise

Tanisha (American)
a combination of the
prefix Ta + Nisha.
Tahniscia, Tahnisha,
Tanicha, Taniesha, Tanish,

Tanisha *(cont.)*
Tanishah, Tanishia,
Tanitia, Tannicia,
Tannisha, Tenisha,
Tenishka, Tinisha,
Tonisha, Tonnisha,
Tynisha

Tanya (Russian, Slavic)
fairy queen. A short form
of Tatiana.
Tahnee, Tahnya, Tana,
Tanaya, Taneya, Tania,
Tanis, Taniya, Tanka,
Tannis, Tanoya, Tany,
Tanyia, Taunya, Tawnya,
Thanya

Tara (Aramaic) throw;
carry. (Irish) rocky hill.
(Arabic) a measurement.
Taira, Tairra, Taraea,
Tarah, Taráh, Tarai,
Taralee, Tarali, Taralyn,
Taran, Tarasa, Tarasha,
Taraya, Tarha, Tari, Tarra,
Taryn, Tayra, Tehra

Tarra (Irish) an alternate
form of Tara.
Tarrah

Taryn (Irish) an alternate
form of Tara.
Taran, Tareen, Tareena,
Taren, Tarene, Tarin,
Tarina, Tarren, Tarrena,
Tarrin, Tarron, Tarryn,
Taryna

Tasha (Greek) born on
Christmas day. (Russian)
a short form of Natasha.
See also Tosha.

Tacha, Tachia, Tachiana,
Tachika, Tahsha, Tasenka,
Tashana, Tashia, Tasia,
Taska, Thasha, Tysha

Tashia (Slavic) a form
of Tasha. (Hausa) a bird
in flight.
Tashi, Tashiana, Tashina

Tasia (Slavic) a familiar
form of Tasha.
Tasiya, Tassi, Tassia,
Tassiana, Tassie, Tasya

Tatiana (Slavic) fairy
queen. See also Tanya,
Tiana.
Taitiann, Taitianna, Tata,
Tatania, Tatanya, Tati,
Tatia, Tatie, Tatihana,
Tatjana, Tatyana,
Tatyanah, Tatyanna,
Tiana, Tiatiana

Tatum (English) cheerful.
Tate, Tatumn

Tavia (Latin) a short form
of Octavia.
Taiva, Tauvia, Tava, Tavah,
Tavie, Tavita

Tawny (Gypsy) little one.
(English) brownish yellow,
tan.
Tahnee, Tany, Tauna,
Tauné, Tauni, Taunia,
Taunisha, Tawna, Tawnee,
Tawnesha, Tawney, Tawni,
Tawnia, Tawnie, Tawnyell,
Tiawna, Tiawni

Tawnya (American)
a combination of
Tawny + Tonya.

Taylor (English) tailor.
Tailor, Taiylor, Talor,
Talora, Taye, Tayla, Taylar,
Tayler, Tayllor, Taylore

Tegan (Welsh) beautiful,
attractive.
Taegen, Teagan, Teaghen,
Teegan, Teeghan, Tega,
Tegan, Teghan, Tegin,
Tegwen, Teigan, Tejan,
Tiegan, Tigan, Tijan,
Tijana

Tenesha, Tenisha
(American) combinations
of the prefix Te + Niesha.
Tenecia, Teneesha,
Teneisha, Tenesha,
Teneshia, Tenesia,
Tenessa, Teneusa,
Tenezya, Teniesha

Tennille (American)
a combination of the
prefix Te + Nellie.
Taniel, Tanille, Teneal,
Teneil, Teneille, Teniel,
Tenille, Tenneal, Tenneill,
Tenneille, Tennia, Tennie,
Tennielle, Tennile, Tineal,
Tiniel, Tonielle, Tonille

Tera, Terra (Latin) earth.
(Japanese) swift arrow.
Teria, Terria

Teresa (Greek) reaper.
An alternate form of
Theresa. See also Tressa.
Taresa, Tarese, Taress,
Taressa, Taris, Tarisa,
Tarise, Tarissa, Teca,
Terasa, Tercza, Tereasa,

Tereatha, Tereese, Tereka,
Terese, Teresea, Teresha,
Teresia, Teresina, Teresita,
Tereska, Tereson, Teress,
Teressa, Teretha, Terez,
Tereza, Terezia, Terezie,
Terezilya, Terezinha,
Terezka, Terezsa, Teri,
Teris, Terisa, Terisha,
Teriza, Terrasa, Terresa,
Terresia, Terrosina, Tersa,
Teruska, Terza, Teté

Teri (Greek) reaper.
A familiar form of Theresa.
Terie

Terri (Greek) reaper.
A familiar form of Theresa.
Terree, Terria, Terrie

Terri-Lynn (American)
a combination of
Terri + Lynn.
Terelyn, Terelynn,
Terrilynn, Terrylynn

Terry (Greek) a short form
of Theresa.
Tere, Teree, Terelle,
Terene, Teri, Terie, Terrey,
Terri, Terrie, Terrye, Tery

Tess (Greek) a short form
of Theresa.

Tessa (Greek) reaper.
A short form of Theresa.
Tesa, Tesha, Tesia, Tessia,
Tezia

Thanh (Vietnamese) bright
blue. (Punjabi) good place.
Thantra, Thanya

Thao (Vietnamese) respect-
ful of parents.

Thea (Greek) goddess.
See also Dorothy.
Theo

Theresa (Greek) reaper.
See also Tracey, Tracy.
**Teresa, Terri, Terry, Tess,
Tessa, Tessie, Theresina,
Theresita, Theressa,
Thereza, Thersa, Thersea,
Tresha, Tressa, Trice**

Therese (Greek) an alter-
nate form of Theresa.
**Terese, Terise, Terrise,
Thérèse, Theresia,
Theressa, Therra,
Therressa, Thersa**

Thi (Vietnamese) poem.
Thia, Thy, Thya

Tia (Greek) princess.
(Spanish) aunt.
**Ti, Téa, Teah, Teeya,
Teia, Tiaisha, Tiajuanna,
Tiakeisha, Tialeigh,
Tiamarie, Tianda,
Tiandria, Tianeka,
Tianika, Tiante,
Tiashauna, Tiawanna, Tiia**

Tiana (Greek) princess.
(Latin) a short form of
Tatiana.
**Teana, Teanna, Tia,
Tiahna, Tianna, Tiaon**

Tiara (Latin) crowned.
**Teair, Teaira, Teairra,
Teara, Téare, Tearra,
Tearia, Tearria, Teearia,
Teira, Teirra, Tiaira,**
**Tiairra, Tiarra, Tiera,
Tiéra, Tierra, Tierre,
Tierrea, Tierria, Tyara,
Tyarra**

Tierney (Irish) noble.
Tiernan

Tiffani, Tiffanie (Latin)
alternate forms of Tiffany.
**Tephanie, Tifanee, Tifani,
Tifanie, Tiff, Tiffanee,
Tiffayne, Tiffeni, Tiffenie,
Tiffennie, Tiffiani,
Tiffianie, Tiffine, Tiffini,
Tiffinie, Tiffni, Tiffy,
Tiffynie, Tifni, Tiphani,
Tiphanie**

Tiffany (Greek) God's
appearance. (Latin) trinity.
**Taffanay, Taffany, Tifaney,
Tifany, Tiff, Tiffaney,
Tiffani, Tiffanie, Tiffanny,
Tiffeney, Tiffiany, Tiffiney,
Tiffiny, Tiffnay, Tiffney,
Tiffny, Tiffy, Tiphany,
Triffany**

Tina (Spanish, American)
a short form of Martina,
Christina, Valentina.
**Teanna, Teena, Teina,
Tena, Tenae, Tine, Tinnia,
Tyna, Tynka**

Tisha (Latin) joy. A short
form of Leticia.
**Taesha, Tesha, Teisha,
Tiesha, Tieshia, Tish,
Tishal, Tishia, Tysha,
Tyshia**

Toni (Greek) flourishing.
(Latin) praiseworthy.

A short form of
Antoinette, Antonia.
**Tonee, Toney, Tonia,
Tonie, Tony**

Tonia (Latin, Slavic)
an alternate form of Toni,
Tonya.
**Tonja, Tonje, Tonna,
Tonni, Tonnia, Tonnie,
Tonnja**

Tonya (Slavic) fairy queen.
Tonia, Tonnya, Tonyetta

Tori (Japanese) bird.
(English) an alternate
form of Tory.
**Toria, Toriana, Torie,
Torri, Torria, Torrie,
Torrina, Torrita**

Tory (Latin) a short form
of Victoria. (English)
victorious.
**Torey, Tori, Torrey,
Torreya, Torrye, Torya,
Torye, Toya**

Tosha (Punjabi) arma-
ments. (Polish) a familiar
form of Antonia. (Russian)
an alternate form of Tasha.
**Toshea, Toshia, Toshiea,
Toshke, Tosia, Toska**

Toya (Spanish) a form
of Tory.
**Toia, Toyanika, Toyanna,
Toyea, Toylea, Toyleah,
Toylenn, Toylin, Toylyn**

Tracey (Greek) a familiar
form of Theresa. (Latin)
warrior.

**Trace, Tracee, Tracell,
Traci, Tracie, Tracy, Traice,
Trasey, Treesy**

Traci, Tracie (Latin) alter-
nate forms of Tracey.
**Tracia, Tracilee, Tracilyn,
Tracilynn, Tracina, Traeci**

Tracy (Greek) a familiar
form of Theresa. (Latin)
warrior.
Treacy

Tressa (Greek) a short
form of Theresa.
**Treaser, Tresa, Tresca,
Trese, Tresha, Treska,
Tressia, Tressie, Trez,
Treza, Trisa**

Trice (Greek) a short form
of Theresa.
Treece

Tricia (Latin) an alternate
form of Trisha.
**Trica, Tricha, Trichelle,
Tricina, Trickia**

Trina (Greek) pure. A short
form of Katrina. (Hindi)
points of sacred kusa
grass.
**Treena, Treina, Trenna,
Triana, Trinia, Trinchen,
Trind, Trinda, Trine,
Trinette, Trinica, Trinice,
Triniece, Trinika, Trinique,
Trinisa, Trinnette, Tryna**

Trisha (Latin) noblewoman.
A familiar form of Patricia.
(Hindi) thirsty. See also
Tricia.

Trisha *(cont.)*
Treasha, Trish, Trishann,
Trishanna, Trishanne,
Trishara, Trishia, Trishna,
Trissha

Trista (Latin) a short form
of Tristen.
Trisatal, Tristess, Tristia,
Trysta, Trystia

Tristen (Latin) bold. A fem-
inine form of Tristan.
Trista, Tristan, Tristian,
Tristiana, Tristin, Tristina,
Tristine, Trystan

Trudy (German) beloved
warrior.
Truda, Trude, Trudessa,
Trudey, Trudi, Trudie

Twyla (English) woven
of double thread.
Twila, Twilla

Tyesha (American)
a combination of the
prefix Ty + Aisha.
Tyisha

Tyler (English) tailor.
Tyller, Tylor

Tyra (Scandinavian) battler.
Mythology: Tyr was the
god of battle.
Tyraa, Tyrah, Tyran,
Tyree, Tyrell, Tyrelle,
Tyrena, Tyrene, Tyresa,
Tyresia, Tyria, Tyrica,
Tyricka, Tyrikka, Tyrina,
Tyronica

U

Ulrica (German) wolf
ruler; ruler of all.
Ulka, Ullrica, Ullricka,
Ullrika, Ulrika, Ulrike

Urika (Omaha) useful
to everyone.

Urit (Hebrew) bright.
Urice

Ursula (Greek) little bear.
Ursa, Ursala, Ursel, Ursela,
Ursella, Ursely, Ursilla,
Ursillane, Ursola, Ursule,
Ursulina, Ursuline,
Urszula, Urszuli, Urzula

V

Valarie (Latin) an alternate
form of Valerie.
Valaria

Valencia (Spanish) strong.
Geography: a region in
eastern Spain.
Valecia, Valence, Valenica,
Valentia, Valenzia

Valene (Latin) a short form
of Valentina.
Valaine, Valean, Valeda,
Valeen, Valen, Valena,
Valeney, Valien, Valina,
Valine, Vallan, Vallen

Valentina (Latin) strong.
History: Valentina
Tereshkova, a Soviet
cosmonaut, was the first
woman in space. See also
Tina, Valene.
Val, Valantina, Vale,
Valentijn, Valentin,
Valentine, Valida, Valtina,
Valyn, Valynn, Velora

Valera (Russian) a form
of Valerie.

Valerie (Latin) strong.
Vairy, Val, Valarae,
Valaree, Valarey, Valari,
Valaria, Valarie, Vale,
Valera, Valeree, Valeri,
Valeria, Valeriana,
Valeriane, Valérie, Valery,
Valerye, Valka, Vallarie,
Valleree, Valleri, Vallerie,
Vallery, Valli, Vallirie,
Valora, Valry, Valya,
Veleria, Velerie, Waleria

Vanessa (Greek) butterfly.
Literature: a name
invented by Jonathan
Swift as a nickname for
Esther Vanhomrigh.
Van, Vanassa, Vanesa,
Vanesha, Vaneshia,
Vanesia, Vanesse,
Vanessia, Vanessica,
Vanetta, Vaneza, Vania,
Vaniece, Vaniessa, Vanija,
Vanika, Vanisa, Vanissa,
Vanita, Vanna, Vannessa,
Vanneza, Vanni, Vannie,
Vanny, Vanya, Varnessa,
Venessa

Vanna (Greek) a short form
of Vanessa. (Cambodian)
golden.
Vana, Vanae, Vannah,
Vannalee, Vannaleigh

Vera (Latin) true. (Slavic)
faith. A short form of
Veronica.
Vara, Veera, Veira,
Veradis, Vere, Verla,
Viera, Vira

Verna (Latin) springtime.
Verne, Vernese, Vernesha,
Verneshia, Vernessa,
Vernetia, Vernetta,
Vernette, Vernia, Vernice,
Vernis, Vernisha,
Vernisheia, Vernita,
Verusya, Viera, Virida,
Virna, Virnell

Veronica (Latin) true
image.
Varonica, Vera, Veranique,
Verenice, Verhonica,
Verinica, Verohnica,
Veron, Verona, Verone,
Veronic, Véronic,
Veronice, Veronika,
Veronique, Véronique,
Veronne, Veronnica,
Vironica, Vonni, Vonnie,
Vonny, Vron, Vronica

Veronique, Véronique
(French) forms of
Veronica.

Vicki (Latin) a familiar form
of Victoria.
**Vic, Vicci, Vicke, Vickee,
Vickiana, Vickie, Vickilyn,
Vickki, Vicky, Vika, Viki,
Vikie, Vikki**

Vicky (Latin) a familiar form
of Victoria.
**Viccy, Vickey, Viky, Vikkey,
Vikky**

Victoria (Latin) victorious.
See also Tory.
**Vicki, Vicky, Victoire,
Victoriana, Victorie,
Victorina, Victorine,
Victory, Viktoria, Vitoria,
Vyctoria**

Violet (French) Botany:
a plant with purplish blue
flowers.
**Vi, Violetta, Violette,
Vyolet, Vyoletta, Vyolette**

Virginia (Latin) pure,
virginal. Literature: Virginia
Woolf was a well-known
British writer. See also
Gina, Ginger, Ginny.
**Verginia, Verginya,
Virge, Virgen, Virgenia,
Virgenya, Virgie, Virgine,
Virginie, Virginië,
Virginio, Virginnia, Virgy,
Virjeana**

Vivian (Latin) full of life.
**Vevay, Vevey, Viv, Viva,
Viveca, Vivee, Vivi, Vivia,**
**Viviana, Viviane, Vivie,
Vivien, Vivienne, Vivina,
Vivion, Vivyan, Vyvyan**

Viviana (Latin) an alternate
form of Vivian.
**Viv, Viviann, Vivianna,
Vivianne, Vivyana,
Vivyann, Vivyanne,
Vyvyana, Vyvyann,
Vyvyanne**

W

Wanda (German) wan-
derer. See also Wendy.
**Vanda, Wahnda, Wandah,
Wandely, Wandi, Wandie,
Wandis, Wandja, Wandy,
Wandzia, Wannda,
Wonda, Wonnda**

Wendi (Welsh) an alternate
form of Wendy.
Wendie

Wendy (Welsh) white; light
skinned. A familiar form of
Gwendolyn, Wanda.
**Wenda, Wende, Wendee,
Wendey, Wendi, Wendye**

Whitney (English) white
island.
**Whiteney, Whitne,
Whitné, Whitnee,
Whitneigh, Whitnie,
Whitny, Whitnye,**

Whittany, Whitteny,
Whittney, Whytne,
Whytney, Witney

Winona (Lakota) oldest
daughter.
Wanona, Wenona,
Wenonah, Winnie,
Winonah, Wynnona,
Wynona

Winter (English) winter.
Wintr, Wynter

Xaviera (Basque) owner
of the new house. (Arabic)
bright. A feminine form
of Xavier.
Xavia, Xavière, Xavyera

Xenia (Greek) hospitable.
See also Zena, Zina.
Xeenia, Xena

Xiang (Chinese) fragrant.

Yasmin, Yasmine (Persian)
alternate forms of Jasmine.

Yashmine, Yasiman,
Yasimine, Yasma,
Yasmain, Yasmaine,
Yasmeen, Yasmene,
Yasmina, Yasminda,
Yasmon, Yasmyn, Yazmen,
Yazmin, Yazmina,
Yazmine, Yesmean,
Yesmeen, Yesmin,
Yesmina, Yesmine,
Yesmyn

Yesenia (Arabic) flower.
Yesnia, Yessena, Yessenia,
Yissenia

Yoko (Japanese) good girl.
Yo

Yolanda (Greek) violet
flower.
Yalanda, Yola, Yolaine,
Yolana, Yoland, Yolande,
Yolane, Yolanna,
Yolantha, Yolanthe,
Yolette, Yolonda,
Yorlanda, Youlanda,
Yulanda, Yulonda

Yuri (Japanese) lily.
Yuriko, Yuriyo

Yvette (French) a familiar
form of Yvonne. See also
Evette, Ivette.
Yavette, Yevett, Yevette,
Yevetta, Yvetta

Yvonne (French) young
archer. (Scandanavian)
yew wood; bow wood.
See also Yvette.
Yavanda, Yavanna,
Yavanne, Yavonda,
Yavonna, Yavonne,

Yvonne (cont.)
Yveline, Yvon, Yvone,
Yvonna, Yvonny

Z

Zacharie (Hebrew) God
remembered. A feminine
form of Zachariah.
Zacari, Zacceaus,
Zacchaea, Zachoia,
Zackeisha, Zackery,
Zakaria, Zakaya,
Zakeshia, Zakiah, Zakir,
Zakiya, Zakiyah, Zechari

Zara (Hebrew) an alternate
form of Sarah, Zora.
Zaira, Zarah, Zaree,
Zareen, Zareena, Zaria

Zelene (English) sunshine.
Zeleen, Zelena, Zeline

Zelia (Spanish) sunshine.
Zele, Zelene, Zelie, Zélie,
Zelina

Zena (Greek) an alternate
form of Xenia. (Ethiopian)
news. (Persian) woman.
See also Zina.
Zeena, Zeenat, Zeenet,
Zeenia, Zeenya, Zein,
Zeina, Zenah, Zenana,
Zenea, Zenia, Zenya

Zina (Greek) an alternate
form of Xenia, Zena.

(African) secret spirit.
(English) hospitable.
Zinah, Zine

Zoe (Greek) life.
Zoé, Zoë, Zoee, Zoelie,
Zoeline, Zoelle, Zoey,
Zoie, Zooey, Zoya

Zora (Slavic) aurora; dawn.
See also Zara.
Zorah, Zorana, Zoreen,
Zoreena, Zorna, Zorra,
Zorrah, Zorya

Zuri (Basque) white;
light skinned. (Swahili)
beautiful.
Zuria, Zurisha

Boys' Names

A

Aaron (Hebrew) enlightened. (Arabic) messenger. Bible: the brother of Moses and the first high priest of the Jews.
Aahron, Aaran, Aaren, Aareon, Aarin, Aaronn, Aarron, Aaryn, Aeron, Aharon, Ahran, Ahren, Aranne, Arek, Aren, Ari, Arin, Aron, Aronek, Aronne, Aronos, Arran, Arron

Abdul (Arabic) servant.
Abdal, Abdeel, Abdel, Abdoul, Abdual, Abul

Abdullah (Arabic) servant of Allah.
Abdalah, Abdalla, Abdallah, Abdualla, Abdulah, Abdulahi

Abel (Hebrew) breath. (Assyrian) meadow. (German) a short form of Abelard. Bible: Adam and Eve's second son.
Abe, Abele, Abell, Able, Adal, Avel

Abraham (Hebrew) father of many nations. Bible: the first Hebrew patriarch. See also Ibrahim.
Abarran, Abe, Aberham, Abey, Abhiram, Abie, Abrahamo, Abrahán, Abrahim, Abrahm, Abram, Abramo, Abrán, Abrao, Arram, Avram

Abram (Hebrew) a short form of Abraham.
Abramo, Abrams, Avram

Adam (Phoenician) man; mankind. (Hebrew) earth; man of the red earth. Bible: the first man created by God. See also Addison.
Ad, Adama, Adamec, Adamo, Adão, Adas, Addam, Addams, Addis, Addy, Adem, Adham, Adhamh, Adné, Adok, Adomas

Addison (English) son of Adam.
Addis, Adison, Adisson

Adham (Arabic) black.

Adrian (Greek) rich. (Latin) dark.
Adarian, Ade, Adorjan, Adrain, Adreian, Adreyan, Adri, Adriaan, Adriane, Adriano, Adrien, Adrik, Adrion, Adron, Adryan, Adryon

Adriel (Hebrew) member of God's flock.
Adrial

Adrien (French) a form of Adrian.
Adriene

Ahmad, Ahmed (Arabic)
most highly praised.
See also Mohammed.
Achmad, Achmed,
Ahamad, Ahamada,
Ahamed, Ahmaad,
Ahmaud, Amad, Amahd,
Amed

Aidan (Irish) fiery.
Aden, Adin, Aiden, Aydan,
Ayden, Aydin

Ajay (Punjabi) victorious;
undefeatable. (American)
a combination of the
initials A. + J.
Aj, Aja, Ajai, Ajaz, Ajit

Akeem (Hebrew) God will
establish. See also Joachim.
Achim, Ackeem, Ackim,
Ahkieme, Akeam, Akee,
Akiem, Akim, Akima,
Arkeem

Alain (French) a form
of Alan.
Alaen, Alainn, Alayn,
Allain

Alan (Irish) handsome;
peaceful.
Ailan, Ailin, Al, Alain,
Alair, Aland, Alani, Alano,
Alanson, Alao, Allan,
Allen, Alon, Alun

Albert (German, French)
noble and bright.
Adelbert, Ailbert, Al,
Albertik, Alberto, Alberts,
Albie, Albrecht, Alvertos,
Aubert

Alberto (Italian) a form
of Albert.
Berto

Alden (English) old; wise
protector.
Aldin, Aldous, Elden

Aldo (Italian) old; elder.

Alec (Greek) a short form
of Alexander.
Aleck, Alek, Alekko, Alic,
Elek

Alejandro (Spanish) a form
of Alexander.
Alejándro, Aléjo,
Alexjándro

Alessandro (Italian) a form
of Alexander.
Alessand, Allessandro

Alex (Greek) a short form
of Alexander.
Alax, Alix, Allax, Allex,
Elek

Alexander (Greek)
defender of mankind.
History: Alexander the
Great was the conquerer
of the Greek Empire.
See also Sandy, Sasha.
Al, Alec, Alecsandar,
Alejandro, Alekos,
Aleksandar, Aleksander,
Aleksandr, Aleksandras,
Aleksandur, Aleksei,
Alessandro, Alex,
Alexandar, Alexandor,
Alexandr, Alexandre,
Alexandros, Alexis,
Alexxander, Alexzander,

Alick, Alisander, Alixander, Alixandre, Lex

Alexandre (French) a form of Alexander.

Alexis (Greek) a short form of Alexander.
Alexei, Alexes, Alexey, Alexi, Alexie, Alexio, Alexios, Alexius, Alexiz, Alexy

Alfonso (Italian, Spanish) a form of Alphonse.
Affonso, Alfons, Alfonse, Alfonsus, Alfonza, Alfonzo, Alfonzus

Alfred (English) elf counselor; wise counselor. See also Fred.
Ailfrid, Ailfryd, Alf, Alfeo, Alfie, Alfredo, Alured

Alfredo (Italian, Spanish) a form of Alfred.
Alfrido

Ali (Arabic) greatest. (Swahili) exalted.
Aly

Allan (Irish) an alternate form of Alan.
Allayne

Allen (Irish) an alternate form of Alan.
Alen, Alley, Alleyn, Alleyne, Allie, Allin, Allon, Allyn

Alonzo (Spanish) a form of Alphonse.

Alano, Alanzo, Alon, Alonso, Alonza, Elonzo, Lon, Lonnie

Alphonse (German) noble and eager.
Alf, Alfie, Alfonso, Alonzo, Alphons, Alphonsa, Alphonso, Alphonsus, Alphonza, Alphonzus, Fonzie

Alphonso (Italian) a form of Alphonse.
Alphanso, Alphonzo, Fonso

Alton (English) old town.
Alten

Alvaro (Spanish) just; wise.

Alvin (Latin) white; light skinned. (German) friend to all; noble friend; friend of elves. See also Elvin.
Aloin, Aluin, Aluino, Alvan, Alven, Alvie, Alvino, Alvy, Alvyn, Alwin, Elwin

Amandeep (Punjabi) light of peace.
Amandip, Amanjit, Amanjot, Amanpreet

Amar (Punjabi) immortal. (Arabic) builder.
Amari, Amario, Amaris, Amarjit, Amarpreet, Ammar, Ammer

Amir (Hebrew) proclaimed. (Punjabi) wealthy; king's minister. (Arabic) prince.
Ameer

Amit (Punjabi) unfriendly.
(Arabic) highly praised.
Amitan, Amreet, Amrit

Ammon (Egyptian) hidden.
Mythology: the ancient
god associated with
reproduction and life.

Amos (Hebrew) burdened,
troubled. Bible: an Old
Testament prophet.

Anders (Swedish) a form
of Andrew.
**Ander, Andersen,
Anderson**

Andre (French) a form
of Andrew.
**Andra, Andrae, André,
Andrecito, Andree,
Andrei, Aundré**

Andreas (Greek) an alternate form of Andrew.
Andrea, Andres, Andries

Andres (Spanish) a form
of Andrew.
Andras, Andrés, Andrez

Andrew (Greek) strong;
manly; courageous.
Bible: one of the Twelve
Apostles. See also Drew.
**Aindrea, Anders, Andery,
Andonis, Andor, András,
André, Andreas, Andrei,
Andres, Andrews, Andru,
Andrue, Andrus, Andy,
Anker, Anndra, Antal,
Audrew**

Andy (Greek) a short form
of Andrew.
Andino, Andis, Andje

Angel (Greek) angel.
(Latin) messenger.
**Ange, Angell, Angelo,
Angie, Angy**

Angelo (Italian) a form
of Angel.
Angelito, Angelos, Anglo

Angus (Scottish) excep-
tional; outstanding.
Mythology: Angus Og was
the Celtic god of laughter,
love, and wisdom.
Aeneas, Aonghas

Anibal (Phoenician) grace
of God.

Anson (German) divine.
(English) Anne's son.
Ansun

Anthony (Latin) praise-
worthy. (Greek) flourish-
ing. See also Tony.
**Anathony, Andonios,
Andor, András, Anothony,
Antal, Antavas, Anfernee,
Anferny, Anthawn,
Anthey, Anthian, Anthino,
Anthoney, Anthoni,
Anthonie, Anthonio,
Anthonu, Anthoy,
Anthyoine, Anthyonny,
Antjuan, Antoine, Anton,
Antonio, Antony, Antwan**

Antoine (French) a form
of Anthony.

**Anntoin, Antionne,
Antoiné, Atoine**

Anton (Slavic) a form
of Anthony.
Antone, Antons, Antos

Antonio (Italian) a form
of Anthony.
**Antinio, Antonello,
Antoino, Antonin,
Antonín, Antonino,
Antonnio, Antonios,
Antonius, Antonyia,
Antonyio, Antonyo**

Antony (Latin) an alternate
form of Anthony.
**Antin, Antini, Antius,
Antoney, Antoni, Antonie,
Antonin, Antonios,
Antonius, Antonyia,
Antonyio, Antonyo, Anty**

Antwan (Arabic) a form
of Anthony.
**Antaw, Antawan,
Antawn, Anthawn,
Antowine, Antowne,
Antowyn, Antwain,
Antwaina, Antwaine,
Antwaion, Antwane,
Antwann, Antwanne,
Antwarn, Antwaun,
Antwen, Antwian,
Antwine, Antwion,
Antwoan, Antwoin,
Antwoine, Antwon,
Antwone, Antwonn,
Antwonne, Antwuan,
Antwyon, Antyon,
Antywon**

Archie (German) bold.
(English) bowman.
Archy

Ari (Hebrew) a short form
of Ariel.
**Aria, Arias, Arie, Arih,
Arij, Ario, Arri**

Aric (German) an alternate
form of Richard. (Scandi-
navian) an alternate form
of Eric.
**Aaric, Areck, Arick, Arik,
Arric, Arrick, Arrik**

Ariel (Hebrew) lion of God.
Bible: another name for
Jerusalem. Literature: the
name of a spirit in the
Shakespearean play
The Tempest.
**Airel, Arel, Areli, Ari,
Ariya, Ariyel, Arrial, Arriel**

Arlen (Irish) pledge.
**Arlan, Arland, Arlend,
Arlin, Arlyn, Arlynn**

Armand (Latin) noble.
(German) soldier. An alter-
nate form of Herman.
**Armad, Arman, Armanda,
Armando, Armands,
Armanno, Armaude,
Armenta, Armond**

Armando (Spanish) a form
of Armand.
Armondo

Arnold (German) eagle
ruler.
**Ardal, Arnald, Arnaldo,
Arnaud, Arne, Arnie,**

Arnold *(cont.)*
Arno, Arnoldo, Arnoll,
Arndt

Aron, Arron (Hebrew)
alternate forms of Aaron.

Arthur (Irish) noble;
lofty hill. (Scottish) bear.
(English) rock. (Icelandic)
follower of Thor.
Art, Artair, Artek, Arth,
Arther, Arthor, Artie,
Artor, Arturo, Artus,
Aurthar, Aurther, Aurthur

Arturo (Italian) a form
of Arthur.
Arthuro, Artur

Asher (Hebrew) happy;
blessed.
Ashar, Ashor, Ashur

Ashley (English) ash-tree
meadow.
Ash, Asheley, Ashelie,
Ashely, Ashlan, Ashleigh,
Ashlen, Ashlie, Ashlin,
Ashling, Ashlinn, Ashlone,
Ashly, Ashlyn, Ashlynn,
Aslan

Ashton (English) ash-tree
settlement.
Ashtin

Aubrey (German) noble;
bearlike. See also Avery.
Aubary, Aube, Aubery,
Aubry, Aubury

August (Latin) a short form
of Augustus.
Agosto, Augie, Auguste,
Augusto

Augustus (Latin) majestic;
venerable. History:
a name used by Roman
emperors such as
Augustus Caesar.
August

Austin (Latin) a short form
of Augustus.
Astin, Austen, Austine,
Auston, Austyn, Oistin,
Ostin

Avery (English) a form
of Aubrey.
Avary, Aveary, Averey,
Averie, Avry

Axel (Latin) axe. (German)
small oak tree; source of
life.
Aksel, Ax, Axe, Axell, Axil,
Axill

B

Baron (German, English)
nobleman, baron.
Baaron, Baronie, Barrion,
Barron, Baryn

Barrett (German) strong
as a bear.
Bar, Baret, Barrat, Barret,
Barrette, Barry

Barry (Welsh) son of Harry.
(Irish) spear, marksman.
(French) gate, fence.

Baris, Barri, Barrie, Barris, Bary

Bart (Hebrew) a short form of Barton.
Barrt, Bartel, Bartie, Barty

Barton (English) barley farm; Bart's town.
Barrton, Bart

Basil (Greek, Latin) royal, kingly. Religion: a saint and leading scholar of the early Christian Church. Botany: an herb used in cooking.
Bas, Base, Baseal, Basel, Basle, Basile, Basilio, Basilios, Basilius, Bassel, Bazek, Bazel, Bazil, Bazyli

Beau (French) handsome.
Beale, Bo

Ben (Hebrew) a short form of Benjamin.
Behn, Benio, Benn, Benne, Benno

Benito (Italian) blessed. History: Benito Mussolini led Italy during World War II.
Benedo, Benino, Benno, Beno, Betto

Benjamin (Hebrew) son of my right hand.
Behnjamin, Bejamin, Bemjiman, Ben, Benejamen, Benejaminas, Beniam, Benja, Benjaim, Benjamaim, Benjaman, Benjamen, Benjamine,

Benjamino, Benjamon, Benjamyn, Benjemin, Benjermain, Benji, Benjie, Benjiman, Benjimen, Benjjmen, Benjy, Benkamin, Benny, Benyamin, Benyamino, Binyamin, Mincho

Bennett (Latin) little blessed one.
Benet, Benett, Bennet

Benny (Hebrew) a familiar form of Benjamin.
Bennie

Benoit (French) a form of Benito. (English) Botany: a yellow, flowering rose plant.

Benson (Hebrew) son of Ben.
Bensen, Benssen, Bensson

Benton (English) Ben's town; town on the moors.
Bent

Bernard (German) brave as a bear. See also Bjorn.
Bear, Bearnard, Benek, Ber, Berend, Bern, Bernabé, Bernadas, Bernal, Bernardel, Bernardin, Bernardo, Bernardus, Bernardyn, Bernarr, Bernat, Bernek, Bernel, Bernerd, Berngards, Bernhard, Bernhards, Bernhardt, Bernie, Bjorn, Burnard

Bert (German, English) bright, shining.
Bertie, Bertus, Birt, Burt

Bilal (Arabic) chosen.
Bila, Billal

Bill (German) a short form of William.
Bil, Billijo, Byll, Will

Billy (German) a familiar form of Bill, William.
Bille, Billey, Billie, Billy, Bily, Willie

Bjorn (Scandinavian) a form of Bernard.
Bjarne

Blaine (Irish) thin, lean. (English) river source.
Blane, Blaney, Blayne, Blayney

Blair (Irish) plain, field. (Welsh) place.
Blaire, Blayr, Blayre

Blaise (Latin) stammerer. (English) flame; trail mark made on a tree.
Ballas, Balyse, Blaisot, Blas, Blase, Blasi, Blasien, Blasius

Blake (English) attractive; dark.
Blakely, Blakeman, Blakey

Blayne (Irish) an alternate form of Blaine.
Blain, Blaine, Blane

Bo (English) a form of Beau.

Bob (English) a short form of Robert.
Bobb, Bobby, Bobek, Rob

Bobby (English) a familiar form of Bob, Robert.
Bobbey, Bobbi, Bobbie, Boby

Boyd (Scottish) yellow haired.
Boid, Boyde

Brad (English) a short form of Bradford, Bradley.
Bradd, Brade

Braden (English) broad valley.
Bradan, Bradden, Bradin, Bradine, Bradyn, Braeden, Braiden, Brayden

Bradford (English) broad river crossing.
Brad, Braddford, Ford

Bradley (English) broad meadow.
Brad, Bradlay, Bradlea, Bradlee, Bradleigh, Bradlie, Bradly, Bradney

Bradly (English) an alternate form of Bradley.

Brady (Irish) spirited. (English) broad island.
Bradey

Branden (English) beacon valley.

Brandon (English) beacon hill.
Bran, Brand, Brandan, Branddon, Brandin, Brandone, Brandonn, Brandyn, Branndan, Brannon

Brandt (English) an alternate form of Brant.

Brant (English) proud.
Brandt, Brannt, Brantley, Brantlie

Braxton (English) Brock's town.

Braydon (English) broad hill.
Bradon, Braedon, Braidon, Brayden

Breck (Irish) freckled.
Brec, Breckie, Brexton

Brendan (Irish) little raven. (English) sword.
Breandan, Bren, Brenden, Brendis, Brendon, Brenn, Brennan, Brenndan, Bryn

Brenden (Irish) an alternate form of Brendan.
Bren, Brendene, Brendin, Brendine

Brennan, Brennen (English, Irish) alternate forms of Brendan.
Bren, Brennin, Brennon

Brent (English) a short form of Brenton.
Brendt, Brentson

Brenton (English) steep hill.
Brent, Brentan, Brenten, Brentin, Brentton, Brentyn

Bret, Brett (Scottish) from Great Britain.

Bhrett, Braten, Braton, Brayton, Breton, Brette, Bretten, Bretton, Brit

Brian (Irish, Scottish) strong; virtuous; honorable. History: Brian Boru was the most famous Irish king.
Briano, Briant, Briante, Brien, Brience, Brient, Brin, Briny, Brion, Bryan

Brice (Welsh) alert; ambitious. (English) son of Rice.
Bricen, Briceton, Bryce

Brit, Britt (Scottish) alternate forms of Bret, Brett.
Brit, Britain, Briton, Brittain, Brittan, Britten, Britton, Brityce

Brock (English) badger.
Broc, Brocke, Brockett, Brockie, Brockley, Brockton, Brocky, Brok, Broque

Broderick (Welsh) son of the famous ruler. (English) broad ridge. See also Roderick.
Brod, Broddie, Broddy, Broderic, Brodric, Brodrick, Brodryck

Brodie (Irish) an alternate form of Brody.
Brodi

Brody (Irish) ditch; canal builder.
Brodee, Broden, Brodey, Brodie, Broedy

Bronson (English) son
of Brown.
**Bransen, Bransin,
Branson, Bron, Bronnie,
Bronnson, Bronny,
Bronsen, Bronsin,
Bronsonn, Bronsson,
Bronsun**

Brook (English) brook,
stream.
**Brooke, Brooker, Brookin,
Brooklyn**

Brooks (English) son
of Brook.
Brookes, Broox

Bruce (French) brushwood
thicket; woods.
Brucey, Brucy, Brue, Bruis

Bruno (German, Italian)
brown haired; brown
skinned.
Brunon, Bruns

Bryan (Irish) strong; virtuous; honorable. An alter-
nate form of Brian.
Bryant, Bryen

Bryant (Irish) an alternate
form of Bryan.
Bryent

Bryce (Welsh) an alternate
form of Brice.
**Brycen, Bryceton, Bryson,
Bryston**

Bryon (German) cottage.
(English) bear.

Bryson (Welsh) son
of Brice.

Buddy (English) herald,
messenger.
Budde, Buddey, Buddie

Byron (French) cottage.
(English) barn.
**Beyren, Beyron, Biren,
Biron, Buiron, Byram,
Byran, Byrann, Byren,
Byrom, Byrone**

C

Cade (Welsh) battler.

Cale (Hebrew) a short form
of Caleb.

Caleb (Hebrew) dog; faith-
ful. (Arabic) bold, brave.
Bible: a companion of
Moses and Joshua.
See also Kaleb.
Caeleb, Calab, Cale, Caley

Calvin (Latin) bald.
See also Kalvin.
Cal, Calv

Camden (Scottish) winding
valley.

Cameron (Scottish)
crooked nose. See also
Kameron.

Cam, Camar, Camaron, Cameran, Camerson, Camiren, Camron

Carey (Greek) pure. (Welsh) castle; rocky island.
Care, Cary

Carl (German) farmer. (English) strong and manly. An alternate form of Charles. A short form of Carlton. See also Kale, Karl.
Carle, Carles, Carless, Carlis, Carll, Carlo, Carlos, Carlson, Carlston, Carlus, Carolos

Carlin (Irish) little champion.
Carlan, Carlen, Carley, Carlie, Carling, Carlino, Carly

Carlo (Italian) a form of Carl, Charles.
Carolo

Carlos (Spanish) a form of Carl, Charles.

Carlton (English) Carl's town.
Carl, Carleton, Carllton, Carlston, Carltonn, Carltton, Charlton

Carmelo (Hebrew) vineyard, garden. See also Carmine.
Carmel, Carmello, Karmel

Carmine (Latin) song; crimson. (Italian) a form of Carmelo.
Carman, Carmen, Carmon

Carr (Scandinavian) marsh.
Karr

Carson (English) son of Carr.
Carrson

Carter (English) cart driver.
Cart

Casey (Irish) brave.
Case, Casie, Casy, Cayse, Caysey, Kacey

Cassidy (Irish) clever; curly haired.
Cass, Cassady, Cassie, Kassidy

Cecil (Latin) blind.
Cece, Cecile, Cecilio, Cecilius, Cecill, Celio, Siseal

Cedric (English) battle chieftain.
Cad, Caddaric, Ced, Cedrec, Cédric, Cedrick, Cedryche, Sedric

Cerek (Greek) an alternate form of Cyril. (Polish) lordly.

Cesar (Spanish) long haired.
Casar, César, Cesare, Cesareo, Cesario, Cesaro

Chad (English) warrior. A short form of Chadwick.

Chad *(cont.)*
Geography: a country
in north-central Africa.
**Ceadd, Chaad, Chadd,
Chaddie, Chaddy, Chade,
Chadleigh, Chadler,
Chadley, Chadlin,
Chadlyn, Chadmen,
Chado, Chadron, Chady**

Chadwick (English)
warrior's town.
Chad, Chadvic, Chadwyck

Chance (English) a short
form of Chauncey.
**Chanc, Chancey, Chancy,
Chanse, Chansy, Chants,
Chantz, Chanz**

Chandler (English)
candle maker.
Chand, Chandlan

Channing (English) wise.
(French) canon; church
official.
Chane, Chann

Charles (German) farmer.
(English) strong and
manly. See also Carl.
**Carlo, Carlos, Charl,
Charle, Charlen, Charlie,
Charlot, Charlzell, Chick,
Chip, Chuck**

Charlie (German, English)
a familiar form of Charles.
Charley, Charly

Chase (French) hunter.
**Chasen, Chason, Chass,
Chasten, Chaston, Chasyn**

Chauncey (English) chan-
cellor; church official.
**Chan, Chance, Chancey,
Chaunce, Chauncei,
Chauncy**

Chaz (English) a familiar
form of Charles.
Chas, Chazwick, Chazz

Chester (English) fortress.
**Ches, Cheslav, Cheston,
Chet**

Chet (English) a short form
of Chester.

Chris (Greek) a short form
of Christian, Christopher.
See also Kris.
**Chriss, Christ, Chrys, Cris,
Crist**

Christian (Greek) follower
of Christ; anointed. See
also Kristian.
**Chretien, Chris, Christa,
Christai, Christain,
Christé, Christen,
Christensen, Christiaan,
Christiana, Christiano,
Christianos, Christin,
Christino, Christion,
Christon, Christos,
Christyan, Chritian,
Chrystian, Cristian,
Crystek**

Christophe (French)
a form of Christopher.
Christoph

Christopher (Greek)
Christ-bearer. Religion:
the patron saint of travel-

ers and drivers. See also
Kristopher.
**Chris, Chrisopherson,
Christafer, Christepher,
Christhoper, Christifer,
Christipher, Christobal,
Christofer, Christoff,
Christoffer, Christofper,
Christoher, Christopehr,
Christoper, Christophe,
Christopherr,
Christophoros,
Christorpher, Christos,
Christovao, Christpher,
Christphere, Christpor,
Christrpher**

Clarence (Latin) clear;
victorious.
**Clarance, Clare, Clarrance,
Clarrence, Clearence**

Clark (French) cleric;
scholar.
Clarke, Clerc, Clerk

Claude (Latin, French)
lame.
**Claud, Claudan, Claudel,
Claudell, Claudian,
Claudianus, Claudien,
Claudin, Claudio, Claudius**

Claudio (Italian) a form
of Claude.

Clay (English) clay pit.
A short form of Clayton.

Clayton (English) town
built on clay.
Clay

Clement (Latin) merciful.
Bible: a disciple of Paul.

**Clem, Clemens, Clément,
Clemente, Clementius,
Clemmons**

Cliff (English) a short form
of Clifford, Clifton.
**Clif, Clift, Clive, Clyff,
Clyph**

Clifford (English) cliff at
the river crossing.
Cliff, Cliford, Clyfford

Clifton (English) cliff town
**Cliff, Cliffton, Clift,
Cliften, Clyfton**

Clint (English) a short
form of Clinton.

Clinton (English) hill town
**Clint, Clinten, Clintton,
Clynton**

Clyde (Welsh) warm.
(Scottish) Geography:
a river in Scotland.
Cly, Clywd

Codey (English) an alternate form of Cody.
Coday

Cody (English) cushion.
History: William Cody
(Buffalo Bill) was a sharp-
shooter and showman in
the American "Wild" West.
See also Kody.
**Code, Codee, Codell,
Codey, Codi, Codiak,
Codie, Coedy**

Colby (English) dark;
dark haired.
Colbey, Collby, Kolby

Cole (Greek) a short form
of Nicholas. (Latin)
cabbage farmer. (English)
a short form of Coleman.
Colet, Coley, Colie

Coleman (Latin) cabbage
farmer. (English) coal
miner.
**Cole, Colemann, Colm,
Colman**

Colin (Greek) a short
form of Nicholas.
(Irish) young cub.
**Cailean, Colan, Cole,
Colen, Collin, Colyn**

Collin (Scottish) a form
of Colin, Collins.
Collen, Collon, Collyn

Collins (Greek) son of
Colin. (Irish) holly.
Collin, Collis

Colt (English) young horse;
frisky. A short form of
Colter, Colton.

Colter (English) herd
of colts.
Colt

Colton (English) coal town.
**Colt, Colten, Coltin,
Coltrane, Kolton**

Connor (Irish) praised,
exalted. (Scottish) wise.
Conner, Conor, Konnor

Conor (Irish) an alternate
form of Connor.

Conrad (German) brave
counselor. See also Konrad.

**Connie, Conrade,
Conrado, Corrado**

Cooper (English) barrel
maker.
Coop, Couper

Corbin (Latin) raven.
**Corban, Corben, Corbey,
Corbie, Corby, Korbin**

Cordell (French) rope
maker.
**Cord, Cordae, Cordale,
Corday, Cordeal, Cordel,
Cordelle, Cordie, Cordy,
Kordell**

Cordero (Spanish) little
lamb.
**Cordaro, Cordeal,
Cordeara, Cordearo,
Cordeiro, Cordelro,
Cordera, Corderall,
Corderro, Corderun,
Cordiaro, Cordy,
Corrderio**

Corey (Irish) hollow.
See also Kory.
**Core, Coreaa, Cori,
Corian, Corie, Corio,
Correy, Corria, Corrie,
Corry, Corrye, Cory**

Cornelius (Greek) cornel
tree. (Latin) horn colored.
**Carnelius, Conny,
Cornealous, Corneili,
Corneilius, Corneliaus,
Cornelious, Cornelis,
Corneliu,Cornell,
Cornellis, Cornellius,
Cornelus, Corney, Cornie,**

Corniellus, Corny,
Cournelius, Nelius, Nellie

Cornell (French) a form
of Cornelius.
Carnell, Cornall, Corney,
Cornie, Corny, Nellie

Corry (Latin) a form of
Corey.

Cortez (Spanish)
conqueror. History:
Hernando Cortez was an
explorer who conquered
the Aztecs in Mexico.
Cartez, Cortes, Courtez

Cory (Latin) a form of
Corey. (French) a familiar
form of Cornell.

Coty (French) slope,
hillside.
Cotee, Cotey, Cotie, Cotty

Courtland (English) court's
land.
Court, Courtlana,
Courtlandt, Courtlin,
Courtlyn

Courtney (English) court.
Cort, Cortnay, Cortne,
Cortney, Court,
Courteney, Courtnay, Curt

Coy (English) woods.
Coyie, Coyt

Craig (Irish, Scottish) crag;
steep rock. See also Kraig.
Crag, Craige, Craigen,
Craigery, Craigon, Creag,
Cregg, Creig, Criag

Cristian (Greek) an alter-
nate form of Christian.
Crétien, Cristhian,
Cristiano, Cristino, Cristle,
Criston, Cristos, Cristy,
Crystek

Cristopher (Greek)
an alternate form of
Christopher.
Cristaph, Cristóbal,
Cristobál, Cristofer,
Cristoph, Cristophe,
Cristoval, Cristovao

Cullen (Irish) handsome.
Cull, Cullan, Cullie, Cullin

Curt (Latin) a short form
of Courtney, Curtis.
See also Kurt.

Curtis (Latin) enclosure.
(French) courteous.
See also Kurtis.
Curio, Currito, Curt,
Curtice, Curtiss, Curtus

Cyril (Greek) lordly.
Cerek, Cerel, Ceril, Ciril,
Cirillo, Cyra, Cyrel, Cyrell,
Cyrelle, Cyrill, Cyrille,
Cyrillus

Cyrus (Persian) sun.
Historial: Cyrus the Great
was a king in ancient
Persia.
Ciro, Cy, Cyris

D

Dakota (Dakota) friend;
partner; tribal name.
**Dac, Dack, Dacoda,
Dacota, DaCota, Dak,
Dakoata, Dakotah,
Dakotha, Dekota, Dekotes**

Dale (English) dale, valley.
**Dael, Dal, Dalen, Daley,
Dalibor, Daly, Dayl, Dayle**

Dallas (Scottish)
Geography: a town in
Scotland; a city in Texas.
**Dal, Dalieass, Dall, Dalles,
Dallis, Dalys, Dellis**

Dalton (English) town in
the valley.
Dal, Dallton, Dalt, Dalten

Damian (Greek) tamer;
soother.
**Daemean, Daemon,
Daemyen, Daimean,
Daimen, Daimon,
Daimyan, Damaiaon,
Dame, Damean,
Dameion, Dameon,
Dameone, Damián,
Damiann, Damiano,
Damianos, Damien,
Damion, Damján,
Damyan, Daymian,
Dema, Demyan**

Damien (Greek) an alternate form of Damian.
Religion: Father Damien
spent his life serving the
leper colony on Molokai
island, Hawaii.
**Daemien, Daimien,
Damie, Damyen**

Damion (Greek) an alter
nate form of Damian.
Damin, Damyon

Damon (Greek) constant,
loyal. (Latin) spirit, demon.
**Daemen, Daemon,
Daemond, Daimon,
Daman, Damen, Damonn,
Damonta, Damontez,
Damontis, Daymon,
Daymond**

Dan (Hebrew) a short
form of Daniel.
(Vietnamese) yes.
Dahn, Danh, Danne

Dana (Scandinavian) from
Denmark.
Dain, Daina

Dane (English) from
Denmark.
**Daine, Danie, Dayne,
Dhane**

Danial (Hebrew) an alter
nate form of Daniel.
Danal, Daneal, Danieal

Daniel (Hebrew) God is
my judge. Bible: a great
Hebrew prophet.
**Dacso, Dan, Daneel,
Daneil, Danek, Danel,**

Danforth, Danial, Dániel, Daniël, Daniele, Danielius, Daniell, Daniels, Danielson, Danila, Danilka, Danilo, Daniyel, Dan'l, Dannel, Danniel, Dannil, Danno, Danny, Danukas, Danyel, Dasco, Dayne, Deniel, Doneal, Doniel, Donois, Dusan, Nelo

Daniele (Hebrew) an alternate form of Daniel.

Danny (Hebrew) a familiar form of Daniel.
Dani, Dannee, Dannie, Dannye, Dany

Dante (Latin) lasting, enduring.
Danatay, Danaté, Dant, Danté, Dauntay, Dauntaye, Daunté, Dauntrae, Deanté, De Anté, Deaunta, Dontae, Donté

Darcy (Irish) dark. (French) from Arcy.
Dar, Daray, D'Aray, Darce, Darcee, Darcel, Darcey, Darcio, D'Arcy, Darsey, Darsy

Darell (English) a form of Darrell.
Daralle, Dareal

Daren (Irish) an alternate form of Darren. (Hausa) born at night.
Dare, Dayren, Dheren

Darin (Irish) an alternate form of Darren.
Darian, Darien, Darion, Darrian, Darrin, Daryn, Darynn, Dayrin, Dearin, Dharin

Darius (Greek) wealthy.
Dairus, Dare, Darieus, Darioush, Darrias, Darrious, Darris, Darrius, Darrus, Derrious, Derris, Derrius

Darnell (English) hidden place.
Dar, Darn, Darnall, Darnel

Daron (Irish) an alternate form of Darren.
Darron, Dayron, Dearon, Dharon, Diron

Darrell (French) darling, beloved; grove of oak trees.
Dare, Darel, Darell, Darral, Darrel, Darrill, Darrol, Darryl, Derrell

Darren (Irish) great. (English) small; rocky hill.
Daran, Dare, Daren, Darin, Daron, Darran, Darrian, Darrien, Darrience, Darrin, Darrion, Darron, Darryn, Darun, Daryn, Dearron, Deren, Dereon, Derren, Derron

Darrick (German) an alternate form of Derek.
Darrec, Darrik, Darryk

Darryl (French) darling, beloved; grove of oak trees. An alternate form of Darrell.
Dahrll, Darryle, Darryll, Daryl, Daryle, Daryll, Derryl

Darwin (English) dear friend. History: Charles Darwin was the naturalist who established the theory of evolution.
Darwyn, Derwin, Derwynn, Durwin

Daryl (French) an alternate form of Darryl.
Darel, Daril, Darl, Darly, Daryell, Daryle, Daryll, Darylle, Daroyl

Dave (Hebrew) a short form of David, Davis.

David (Hebrew) beloved. Bible: the first king of Israel.
Dabi, Daevid, Dafydd, Dai, Daivid, Daoud, Dauid, Dav, Dave, Daved, Daveed, Daven, Davey, Davidde, Davide, Davido, Davon, Davoud, Davyd, Dawid, Dawit, Dawud, Dayvid, Dov

Davin (Scandinavian) brilliant Finn.
Daevin, Davinte, Davon, Dawin, Dawine

Davis (Welsh) son of David.
Dave, Davidson, Davies, Davison

Davon (American) a form of Davin.
Daevon, Davon, Davone, Davonn, Davonne, Davonte, Dayvon, Devon

Dawson (English) son of David.

Dayne (Scandinavian) a form of Dane.

Dayton (English) day town; bright, sunny town.
Daeton, Daiton, Deyton

Dean (French) leader. (English) valley. See also Dino.
Deane, Deen, Dene, Deyn

Deandre (French) a combination of the prefix De + Andre.
D'andre, D'andré, D'André, D'andrea, Deandrae, Déandre, Deandré, Deandra, De André, Deandrea, De Andrea, Deaundera, Deaundra, Deaundre, De Aundre, Deaundrey, Deondray, Deondre, Deondré

Deangelo (Italian) a combination of the prefix De + Angelo.
Dang, Dangelo, D'Angelo, Danglo, Deaengelo, Déangelo, De Angelo, Deangleo, Deanglo, Diangelo, Di'angelo

Dejuan (American)
a combination of the
prefix De + Juan.
**Dejan, Dejon, Dejun,
Dewan, Dewaun, Dewon,
Dijaun, D'Juan, Dujuan,
D'Won**

Delbert (English) bright as
day.
Bert, Del, Dilbert

Delvin (English) proud
friend; friend from the
valley.
**Del, Delavan, Delvyn,
Delwin**

Demarco (Italian)
a combination of the
prefix De + Marco.
Damarco, D'Marco

Demarcus (American)
a combination of the
prefix De + Marcus.
**Damarcius, Damarcus,
Demarkes, Demarkis,
Demarkus, D'Marcus**

Demario (Italian)
a combination of the
prefix De + Mario.
**Demarreio, Demarrio,
Demerrio**

Demetris (Greek) a short
form of Demetrius.
**Demeatric, Demeatrice,
Demeatris, Demetres,
Demetress, Demetric,
Demetrice, Demetrick,
Demetrics, Demetricus,
Demetrik, Demitrez**

Demetrius (Greek) lover
of the earth. Mythology:
a follower of Demeter, the
goddess of the harvest and
fertility. See also Dimitri.
**Damitriuz, Demeitrius,
Demeterious, Demetreus,
Demetrias, Demetrio,
Demetrios, Demetrious,
Demetris, Demetriu,
Demetrium, Demetrois,
Demetruis, Demetrus,
Demitirus, Demitri,
Demitrias, Demitriu,
Demitrius, Demitrus,
Demtrius, Demtrus,
Dimitri, Dimitrios,
Dimitrius, Dmetrius,
Dymek**

Denis (Greek) an alternate
form of Dennis.

Dennis (Greek) Mythology:
a follower of Dionysius,
the god of wine. See also
Dion.
**Den, Dénes, Denies, Denis,
Deniz, Dennes, Dennet,
Denny, Dennys, Denya,
Denys, Deon, Dinis**

Denny (Greek) a familiar
form of Dennis.
**Den, Denney, Dennie,
Deny**

Denver (English) green
valley. Geography:
the capital of Colorado.

Deon (Greek) an alternate form of Dennis. See also Dion.
Deion, Deone, Deonno

Derek (German) ruler of the people. See also Dirk.
Darek, Darick, Darrick, Derak, Dereck, Derecke, Derele, Derick, Derk, Derke, Derrek, Derrick, Deryek

Derick (German) an alternate form of Derek.
Deric, Dericka, Derico, Deriek, Derik, Derikk, Derique, Deryck, Deryk, Deryke, Detrek

Deron (Hebrew) bird; freedom. (American) a combination of the prefix De + Ron.
Daaron, Daron, Da-Ron, Darone, Darron, Dayron, Dereon, Deronn, Deronne, Derrin, Derrion, Derron, Derronn, Derronne, Derryn, Diron, Duron, Durron, Dyron

Derrek (German) an alternate form of Derek.
Derrec, Derreck

Derrell (French) an alternate form of Darrell.
Derrel, Dérrell, Derriel, Derril, Derrill

Derrick (German) ruler of the people. An alternate form of Derek.

Derric, Derrik, Derryck, Derryk

Deshawn (American) a combination of the prefix De + Shawn.
Dasean, Dashaun, Dashawn, Desean, Deshaun, Deshaune, Deshauwn, Deshawan, D'Sean, D'shaun, D'Shaun, D'shawn, D'Shawn, Dusean, Dushan, Dushaun, Dushawn

Desmond (Irish) from south Munster.
Demond, Des, Desi, Desmon, Desmund, Dezmon, Dezmond

Deven (Hindi) for God. (Irish) an alternate form of Devin.
Deaven, Deiven

Devin (Irish) poet.
Deavin, Deivin, Dev, Devan, Deven, Devlyn, Devy, Dyvon

Devon (Irish) an alternate form of Devin.
Deavon, Deivon, Deivone, Deivonne, Devoen, Devohn, Devone, Devonn, Devonne, Devontae, Devontaine, Devontay, Devyn

Dewayne (Irish) an alternate form of Dwayne. (American) a combination of the prefix De + Wayne.

Deuwayne, Devayne, Dewain, Dewaine, Dewan, Dewon, Dewune

Dewey (Welsh) prized.
Dew, Dewi, Dewie

Dexter (Latin) dexterous, adroit. (English) fabric dyer.
Daxter, Decca, Deck, Decka, Dekka, Dex, Dextar, Dextor, Dextrel, Dextron

Diego (Spanish) a form of Jacob, James.
Diaz, Iago, Jago

Dillon (Irish) loyal, faithful. See also Dylan.
Dil, Dilan, Dill, Dillan, Dillen, Dillie, Dillin, Dillion, Dilly, Dillyn, Dilon, Dilyn

Dimitri (Russian) a form of Demetrius.
Dimetra, Dimetri, Dimetric, Dimetrie, Dimitr, Dimitric, Dimitrie, Dimitrik, Dimitris, Dimitry, Dimmy, Dmitri, Dymitr, Dymitry

Dimitrios (Greek) an alternate form of Demetrius.
Dhimitrios, Dimitrius, Dimos, Dmitrios

Dino (German) little sword. (Italian) a form of Dean.
Deano

Dion (Greek) a short form of Dennis.

Deon, Dio, Dione, Dionigi, Dionis, Dionn, Diontae, Dionte, Diontray

Dirk (German) a short form of Derek.
Derk, Dirck, Dirke, Durc, Durk, Dyrk

Domenico (Italian) a form of Dominic.
Domenic, Domicio, Dominico, Menico

Dominic (Latin) belonging to the Lord.
Deco, Demenico, Dom, Domanic, Domeka, Domenic, Domenico, Domini, Dominie, Dominique, Dominitric, Dominy, Domnenique, Domonic, Nick

Dominick (Latin) an alternate form of Dominic.
Domenick, Domiku, Domineck, Dominick, Dominicke, Dominiek, Dominik, Domminick, Domnick, Domokos, Domonick, Donek, Dumin

Dominique (French) a form of Dominic.
Domeniqu, Domenque, Dominiqu, Dominiqueia, Domnenique, Domnique, Domoniqu, Domonique

Don (Scottish) a short form of Donald.
Donn

Donald (Scottish) world leader; proud ruler.
Don, Donal, Dónal, Donaldo, Donall, Donalt, Donát, Donaugh, Donnie

Donnell (Irish) brave; dark.
Doneal, Donell, Donelle, Donnelly, Doniel, Donielle, Donnel, Donnelle, Donniel

Donnie, Donny (Irish) familiar forms of Donald.

Donovan (Irish) dark warrior.
Dohnovan, Donavan, Donavin, Donavon, Donavyn, Donevon, Donoven, Donovin, Donovon, Donvan

Dontae, Donté (American) forms of Dante.
Donta, Dontai, Dontao, Dontate, Dontay, Dontaye, Dontea, Dontee, Dontez

Dorian (Greek) from Doris, Greece.
Dore, Dorey, Dorie, Dorien, Dorion, Dorján, Dorrian, Dorrien, Dorryen, Dory

Douglas (Scottish) dark river, dark stream.
Doug, Douglass, Dougles, Dugaid, Dughlas

Doyle (Irish) dark stranger.
Doy, Doyal, Doyel

Drake (English) dragon; owner of the inn with the dragon trademark.
Drago

Drew (Welsh) wise. (English) a short form of Andrew.
Drewe, Dru

Duane (Irish) an alternate form of Dwayne.
Deune, Duain, Duaine, Duana

Duncan (Scottish) brown warrior. Literature: King Duncan was MacBeth's victim in Shakespeare's play *MacBeth*.
Dunc, Dunn

Durell (Scottish, English) king's doorkeeper.
Dorrell, Durel, Durial, Durreil, Durrell, Durrelle

Dustin (German) valiant fighter. (English) brown rock quarry.
Dust, Dustan, Dusten, Dustie, Dustine, Duston, Dusty, Dustyn

Dusty (English) a familiar form of Dustin.

Dustyn (English) an alternate form of Dustin.

Dwayne (Irish) dark. See also Dewayne.
Dawayne, Dawyne, Duane, Duwain, Duwan, Duwane, Duwayn, Duwayne, Dwain, Dwaine,

Dwan, Dwane, Dwyane, Dywane

Dwight (English) blond.

Dylan (Welsh) sea. See also Dillon.
Dyllan, Dyllon, Dylon

E

Earl (Irish) pledge. (English) nobleman.
Airle, Earld, Earle, Earlie, Earlson, Early, Eorl, Erl, Erle, Errol

Earnest (English) an alternate form of Ernest.
Earn, Earnesto, Earnie, Eranest

Eddie (English) a familiar form of Edgar, Edward.
Eddee, Eddy

Eddy (English) an alternate form of Eddie.
Eddye, Edy

Edgar (English) successful spearman.
Ed, Eddie, Edek, Edgard, Edgardo, Edgars

Edmond (English) an alternate form of Edmund.
Eamon, Edmon, Edmonde, Edmondo, Edmondson, Esmond

Edmund (English) prosperous protector.
Eadmund, Eamon, Edmond, Edmundo, Edmunds

Eduardo (Spanish) a form of Edward.

Edward (English) prosperous guardian. See also Ted, Teddy.
Ed, Eddie, Edik, Edko, Edo, Edoardo, Edorta, Édouard, Eduard, Eduardo, Edus, Edvard, Edvardo, Edwardo, Edwards, Edwy, Edzio, Ekewaka, Etzio, Ewart

Edwin (English) prosperous friend.
Eadwinn, Edik, Edlin, Eduino, Edwyn

Efrain (Hebrew) fruitful.
Efrane

Elam (Hebrew) highlands.

Eldon (English) holy hill.

Eli (Hebrew) uplifted. A short form of Elijah, Elisha. Bible: the high priest who trained the prophet Samuel. See also Elliot.
Elie, Elier, Eloi, Eloy, Ely

Elias (Greek) a form of Elijah.
Elia, Eliasz, Elice, Ellice, Ellis, Elyas

Elijah (Hebrew) the Lord is
my God. Bible: a great
Hebrew prophet. See also
Eli, Elisha, Elliot.
**El, Elia, Elias, Elija, Elijuo,
Elisjsha, Eliya, Eliyahu,
Ellis**

Elisha (Hebrew) God is my
salvation. Bible: a great
Hebrew prophet, succes-
sor to Elijah. See also Eli.
**Elijsha, Elisee, Elisée,
Eliseo, Elish, Elisher,
Elishia, Elishua, Lisha**

Elliot, Elliott (English)
forms of Eli, Elijah.
**Elio, Eliot, Eliott, Eliud,
Eliut, Elyot, Elyott**

Ellis (English) a form
of Elias.

Elmer (English) noble;
famous.
**Aylmer, Elemér, Ellmer,
Elmir, Elmo**

Elton (English) old town.
Alton, Eldon, Ellton

Elvin (English) a form
of Alvin.
**El, Elvyn, Elwin, Elwyn,
Elwynn**

Elvis (Scandinavian) wise.
El, Elvys

Emanuel (Hebrew)
an alternate form
of Emmanuel.
**Emaniel, Emanual,
Emanuele**

Emerson (German, English)
son of Emery.
Emmerson, Emreson

Emery (German) industri-
ous leader.
**Emari, Emeri, Emerich,
Emerio, Emmerich,
Emmerie, Emmery, Emmo,
Emory, Imre, Imrich**

Emil (Latin) flatterer.
(German) industrious.
**Aymil, Émile, Emilek,
Emiliano, Emilio, Emill,
Emils, Emilyan, Emlyn**

Emilio (Italian, Spanish)
a form of Emil.
Emilio, Emilios, Emilo

Emmanuel (Hebrew)
God is with us. See also
Manuel.
**Eman, Emanuel, Emanuell,
Emek, Emmaneuol,
Emmanle, Emmanueal,
Emmanuele, Emmanuil**

Emmett (German) industri-
ous; strong. (English) ant.
History: Robert Emmett
was an Irish patriot.
**Em, Emitt, Emmet, Emmit,
Emmot, Emmott, Emmy**

Emory (German) an alternate form of Emery.
Emmory, Emrick

Enrique (Spanish) a form
of Henry.
**Enrigué, Enriqué,
Enriquez, Enrrique**

Eric (German) a short form of Frederick. (Scandinavian) ruler of all. (English) brave ruler. History: Eric the Red was a Norse hero and explorer. See also Aric.
Ehrich, Elika, Erek, Éric, Erica, Erich, Erick, Erickson, Erico, Ericson, Erik, Erric, Eryc, Eryk, Rick

Erich (Czech, German) a form of Eric.

Erik (Scandinavian) an alternate form of Eric.
Erek, Eriks, Erikson, Erikur, Errick

Erin (Irish) peaceful. History: another name for Ireland.
Erine, Erinn, Erino, Eryn, Erynn

Ernest (English) earnest, sincere.
Earnest, Ernestino, Ernesto, Ernestus, Ernie, Erno, Ernst

Ernesto (Spanish) a form of Ernest.
Ernester, Neto

Errol (Latin) wanderer. (English) an alternate form of Earl.
Erol, Erold, Erroll, Erryl

Ervin, Erwin (English) sea friend. See also Irving.
Earvin, Erv, Erven, Ervyn, Erwan, Erwinek, Erwinn, Erwyn, Erwynn

Esteban (Spanish) a form of Stephen.
Estabon, Estefan, Estephan

Ethan (Hebrew) strong; firm.
Eathan, Etan, Ethe

Eugene (Greek) born to nobility. See also Gene, Gino, Yevgenyi.
Eoghan, Eugen, Eugéne, Eugeni, Eugenio, Eugenius, Evgeny, Ezven

Evan (Irish) young warrior. (English) a form of John. See also Keon, Owen.
Eoin, Ewan, Ewen, Ev, Evann, Evans, Even, Evens, Evin, Evyn

Everett (German) courageous as a boar.
Ev, Evered, Everet, Everette, Everitt, Evert, Evrett

Ezekiel (Hebrew) strength of God. Bible: a Hebrew prophet.
Ezéchiel, Ezeck, Ezeeckel, Ezekeial, Ezekial, Ezell, Ezequiel, Eziakah, Eziechiele, Eziequel

Ezra (Hebrew) helper; strong. Bible: a prophet and leader of the Israelites.
Esdras, Esra, Ezer, Ezera, Ezri

F

Fabian (Latin) bean
grower.
Fabayan, Fabe, Fabek,
Fabeon, Faber, Fabert,
Fabi, Fabiano, Fabien,
Fabio, Fabius, Fabiyan,
Fabiyus, Fabyan, Fabyen,
Faybian, Faybien

Fabio (Latin) an alternate
form of Fabian.

Felipe (Spanish) a form
of Philip.
Feeleep, Felipino, Felo,
Filip, Filippo, Filips, Fillip,
Flip

Felix (Latin) fortunate;
happy.
Fee, Felic, Félice, Feliciano,
Felicio, Felike, Feliks, Felo,
Félix, Felizio, Phelix

Ferdinand (German)
daring, adventurous.
Ferdie, Ferdynand,
Fernando, Nando

Fernando (Spanish) a form
of Ferdinand.
Ferdinando Ferdnando,
Ferdo, Fernand,
Fernandez

Fletcher (English) arrow
featherer, arrow maker.
Flecher, Fletch

Floyd (English) a form
of Lloyd.

Forest (French) an alternate form of Forrest.

Forrest (French) forest;
woodsman.
Forest, Forester, Forrie

Francesco (Italian) a form
of Francis.

Francis (Latin) free;
from France. Religion:
Saint Francis of Assisi
was the founder of
the Franciscan order.
Fran, France, Francessco,
Franchot, Francisco,
Franciskus, François,
Frang, Frank, Frannie,
Franny, Frans, Franscis,
Fransis, Franta, Frantisek,
Frants, Franus, Franz,
Frantisek, Frencis

Francisco (Portuguese,
Spanish) a form of Francis.
Franco, Fransisco, Frasco,
Frisco

François (French) a form
of Francis.

Frank (English) a short
form of Francis, Franklin
Franc, Franck, Franek,
Frang, Franio, Franke,
Frankie, Franko

Frankie (English) a familiar
form of Frank.
Franky

Franklin (English) free
landowner.
**Fran, Francklin, Francklyn,
Frank, Frankin, Franklinn,
Franklyn, Franquelin**

Franklyn (English) an alternate form of Franklin.
Franklynn

Fraser (French) strawberry.
(English) curly haired.
**Fraizer, Frasier, Fraze,
Frazer, Frazier**

Fred (German) a short form
of Frederick. See also
Alfred.
Fredd, Fredo, Fredson

Freddie (German) a famil-
iar form of Frederick.
**Freddi, Freddy, Fredi,
Fredy**

Frederick (German) peace-
ful ruler. See also Eric.
**Federico, Fico, Fred,
Fredderick, Freddie,
Freddrick, Fredek,
Fréderick, Frédérick,
Frederik, Frédérik,
Frederrick, Fredo,
Fredrick, Fredrik,
Fredwick, Fredwyck,
Friedrich, Fritz**

Fredrick (German) an
alternate form of
Frederick.

**Frederic, Frédéric,
Frederich, Frederric,
Fredric, Fredrich**

Fritz (German) a familiar
form of Frederick.
**Fritson, Fritts, Fritzchen,
Fritzl**

G

Gabriel (Hebrew) devoted
to God. Bible: the
Archangel of
Annunciation.
**Gab, Gabe, Gabby,
Gaberial, Gabin, Gabino,
Gabis, Gábor, Gabrail,
Gabreil, Gabriël, Gabriele,
Gabriell, Gabrielli, Gabris,
Gabys, Gavril, Gebereal,
Ghabriel, Riel**

Galen (Greek) healer; calm.
(Irish) little and lively.
**Gaelan, Gaelen, Galan,
Gale, Galeno, Galin,
Gaylen**

Gareth (Welsh) gentle.
**Gar, Garith, Garreth,
Garth, Garyth**

Garett (Irish) an alternate
form of Garrett.
Gared, Garet

Garrett (Irish) brave
spearman. See also Jarrett

Garrett (cont.)
**Gar, Gareth, Garett,
Garrad, Garret, Garrette,
Gerret, Gerrett, Gerrit,
Gerritt, Gerrot, Gerrott**

Garrison (French) troops
stationed at a fort;
garrison.
Garris

Garry (English) an alternate
form of Gary.
**Garrey, Garri, Garrie,
Garrin**

Garth (Scandinavian)
garden, gardener. (Welsh)
a short form of Gareth.

Gary (German) mighty
spearman. (English) a
familiar form of Gerald.
Gare, Garey, Gari, Garry

Gavin (Welsh) white hawk.
**Gav, Gavan, Gaven,
Gavinn, Gavino, Gavyn,
Gavynn, Gawain**

Gene (Greek) born to
nobility. A short form
of Eugene.
Genek

Geoffrey (English) divinely
peaceful. A form of Jeffrey.
See also Jeff.
**Geffrey, Geoff, Geoffery,
Geoffre, Geoffroi,
Geoffroy, Geoffry,
Geofrey, Geofri, Gofery**

George (Greek) farmer.
See also Jorge.

**Geordie, Georg, Georgas,
Georges, Georget, Georgi,
Georgii, Georgio,
Georgios, Georgiy,
Georgy, Gevork,
Gheorghe, Giorgio,
Giorgos, Goerge, Goran,
Gordios, Gorge, Gorje,
Gorya, Grzegorz, Gyorgy**

Gerald (German) mighty
spearman. See also Jarell,
Jarrell, Jerald, Jerry.
**Garald, Garold, Garolds,
Gary, Gearalt, Gellert,
Gérald, Geralde, Geraldo,
Gerale, Geraud, Gerek,
Gerick, Gerik, Gerold,
Gerrald, Gerrell, Gérrick,
Gerrild, Gerrin, Gerrit,
Gerrold, Gerry, Geryld,
Giraldo, Giraud, Girauld**

Gerard (English) brave
spearman. See also
Jerrard, Jerry.
**Garrard, Garrat, Garratt,
Gearard, Gerad, Gerar,
Gérard, Gerardo, Geraro,
Géraud, Gerd, Gerek,
Gerhard, Gerrard, Gerrit,
Gerry, Gherardo, Girard**

Gerardo (Spanish) a form
of Gerard.

Gerrit (Dutch) a form
of Gerald.

Gerry (English) a familiar
form of Gerald, Gerard.
See also Jerry.
**Geri, Gerre, Gerri, Gerrie,
Gerryson**

Giancarlo (Italian) a combination of John + Charles.
Giancarlos

Gideon (Hebrew) tree cutter. Bible: the judge who delivered the Israelites from captivity.
Gedeon, Gideone, Gidon, Hedeon

Gilbert (English) brilliant pledge; trustworthy.
Gib, Gilberto, Gilburt, Giselbert, Giselberto, Giselbertus, Guilbert

Gilberto (Spanish) a form of Gilbert.

Gilles (French) goatskin shield.
Gide, Giles, Gyles

Gino (Greek) a familiar form of Eugene. (Italian) a short form of names ending in "gene," "gino."
Ghino

Giovanni (Italian) a form of John.
Geovanni, Gian, Gianni, Giannino, Giavani, Giovani, Giovannie, Giovanno, Giovanny, Giovany, Giovonathon, Giovonni

Giuseppe (Italian) a form of Joseph.
Giuseppino

Glen (Irish) an alternate form of Glenn.
Glyn

Glenn (Irish) woody valley, glen.
Gleann, Glen, Glennie, Glennis, Glennon, Glenny, Glynn

Gordon (English) triangular hill.
Geordan, Gord, Gordain, Gordan, Gorden, Gordy

Grady (Irish) noble; illustrious.
Gradea, Gradee, Gradey, Gradleigh, Graidey, Graidy

Graeme (Scottish) a form of Graham.
Graem

Graham (English) grand home.
Graeham, Graehame, Graehme, Graeme, Grahame, Grahme, Gram

Grant (English) great; giving.
Grand, Grantham, Granthem, Grantley

Grayson (English) bailiff's son. See also Sonny.
Greydon, Greyson

Greg, Gregg (Latin) short forms of Gregory.
Graig, Greig, Gregson

Greggory (Latin) an alternate form of Gregory.
Greggery

Gregory (Latin) vigilant watchman.

Gregory *(cont.)*
**Gergely, Gergo, Greagoir,
Greagory, Greer, Greg,
Gregary, Greger, Gregery,
Greggory, Grégoire,
Gregor, Gregori, Grégorie,
Gregorio, Gregorius,
Gregors, Gregos, Gregrey,
Gregroy, Gregry, Greogry,
Gries, Grisha, Grzegorz**

Griffin (Latin) hooked
nose.
**Griff, Griffen, Griffie,
Griffon, Griffy, Gryphon**

Guillaume (French)
a form of William.
Guillaums

Guillermo (Spanish)
a form of William.

Gurpreet (Punjabi)
devoted to the guru;
devoted to the Prophet.
**Gurjeet, Gurmeet,
Guruprit**

Gustave (Scandinavian)
staff of the Goths. History:
Gustavus Adolphus was a
king of Sweden.
**Gus, Gustaf, Gustaff,
Gustav, Gustavo, Gustus**

Gustavo (Italian, Spanish)
a form of Gustave.

Guy (Hebrew) valley.
(German) warrior. (French)
guide.
Guyon

H

Hakim (Arabic) wise.
(Ethiopian) doctor.
Hakeem, Hakiem

Hank (American) a familiar
form of Henry.

Hans (Scanadinavian)
a form of John.
**Hanschen, Hansel, Hants,
Hanz**

Hardeep (Punjabi) an alternate form of Harpreet.

Harlan (English) hare's
land; army land.
**Harland, Harlen, Harlenn,
Harlin, Harlon, Harlyn,
Harlynn**

Harley (English) hare's
meadow; army meadow.
**Arley, Harlea, Harlee,
Harleigh, Harly**

Harold (Scandinavian)
army ruler.
**Araldo, Garald, Garold,
Hal, Harald, Haraldas,
Haraldo, Haralds, Harry,
Heraldo, Herold, Heronim,
Herrick, Herryck**

Harpreet (Punjabi) loves
God, devoted to God.
Hardeep

Harris (English) a short
form of Harrison.
Haris, Hariss

Harrison (English) son
of Harry.
Harris, Harrisen

Harry (English) a familiar
form of Harold.
**Harm, Harray, Harrey,
Harri, Harrie**

Harvey (German) army
warrior.
Harv, Hervé, Hervey, Hervy

Hassan (Arabic) handsome.
Hasan

Hayden (English) hedged
valley.
**Haden, Haidyn, Haydn,
Haydon**

Heath (English) heath.
Heathe, Heith

Hector (Greek) steadfast.
Mythology: the greatest
hero of the Trojan war.

Henry (German) ruler of
the household. See also
Enrique.
**Hagan, Hank, Harro,
Harry, Heike, Heinrich,
Heinz, Hendrick, Henery,
Heniek, Henning, Henraoi,
Henri, Henrick, Henrim,
Henrique, Henrry,
Heromin, Hersz**

Herbert (German) glorious
soldier.

**Bert, Erbert, Harbert,
Hebert, Hébert, Heberto,
Herb, Heriberto, Hurbert**

Heriberto (Spanish) a form
of Herbert.
Heribert

Herman (Latin) noble.
(German) soldier. See also
Armand.
**Harmon, Hermann,
Hermie, Herminio,
Hermino, Hermon, Hermy,
Heromin**

Hiram (Hebrew) noblest;
exalted.
Hi, Hirom, Huram, Hyrum

Homer (Greek) hostage;
pledge; security. Literature:
a renowned Greek poet.
**Homere, Homère,
Homero, Homeros,
Homerus**

Horace (Latin) keeper
of the hours. Literature:
a famous Latin poet.
Horacio, Horaz

Houston (English) hill
town. Geography:
a city in Texas.
Huston

Howard (English) watchman.
Howie, Ward

Hubert (German) bright
mind; bright spirit.
**Bert, Hobart, Hubbard,
Hubbert, Huber, Huberto,**

Hubert *(cont.)*
Hubie, Huey, Hugh,
Hugibert, Humberto

Hugh (English) a short form
of Hubert.
Fitzhugh, Hew, Hiu, Huey,
Hughes, Hugo, Hugues

Hugo (Latin) a form
of Hugh.
Ugo

Humberto (German)
brilliant strength.

Hunter (English) hunter.
Hunt

Huy (Vietnamese) glorious.

I

Iain (Scottish) an alternate
form of Ian.

Ian (Scottish) a form of
John.
Iain

Ibrahim (Arabic) a form
of Abraham. (Hausa) my
father is exalted.
Ibraham, Ibrahem

Imran (Arabic) host. Bible:
a character in the Old
Testament.

Ira (Hebrew) watchful.

Irvin (Irish, Welsh, English)
a short form of Irving.
Inek, Irv, Irvine

Irving (Irish) handsome
(Welsh) white river.
(English) sea friend.
See also Ervin.
Irv, Irvin, Irvington

Isaac (Hebrew) he will
laugh. Bible: the son of
Abraham and Sarah.
Aizik, Icek, Ike, Ikey, Ikie,
Isaak, Isaakios, Isac, Ishaq,
Isacco, Isack, Isak, Isiac,
Isiacc, Issca, Issiac, Itzak,
Izak, Izzy

Isaiah (Hebrew) God is my
salvation. Bible: an influen-
tial Hebrew prophet.
Isa, Isai, Isaia, Isaid, Isaih,
Isais, Isaish, Ishaq, Isia,
Isiah, Isiash, Issia, Issiah,
Izaiah, Izaiha

Ismael (Hebrew) God will
hear. Literature: the narra-
tor of Melville's novel
Moby Dick.
Isamail, Ishma, Ishmael,
Ishmel, Ismail

Israel (Hebrew) prince of
God; wrestled with God.
History: the nation of Israel
took its name from the
name given Jacob after he
wrestled with the Angel of
the Lord.
Iser, Isser, Izrael, Izzy,
Yisrael

Ivan (Russian) a form of John.
Iván, Ivanchik, Ivanichek, Ivano, Ivas, Vanya

J

J (American) an initial used as a first name.
J.

Jace (American) a combination of the initials J. + C.
JC, J.C., Jacey, Jaice, Jayce, Jaycee

Jack (American) a familiar form of Jacob, John.
Jackie, Jacko, Jackub, Jacque, Jak, Jax, Jock, Jocko

Jackie (American) a familiar form of Jack.
Jacky

Jackson (English) son of Jack.
Jacson, Jakson, Jaxon

Jacob (Hebrew) supplanter, substitute. Bible: son of Abraham, brother of Esau. See also Diego, James, Yakov.
Jaap, Jachob, Jack, Jackub, Jaco, Jacobb, Jacobe, Jacobi, Jacobis, Jacobo, Jacobs, Jacobus, Jacoby, Jacolby, Jacques, Jago, Jaime, Jake, Jakob, Jalu, Jasha, Jecis, Jeks, Jeska, Jim, Jocek, Jock, Jocoby, Jocolby, Jokubas

Jacques (French) a form of Jacob, James.
Jacot, Jacquan, Jacquees, Jacquet, Jacquez, Jaques, Jarques, Jarquis

Jade (Spanish) jade, precious stone.

Jaime (Spanish) a form of Jacob, James.
Jaimey, Jaimie, Jaimito, Jayme, Jaymie

Jake (Hebrew) a short form of Jacob.
Jakie, Jayk, Jayke

Jakob (Hebrew) an alternate form of Jacob.
Jakab, Jakiv, Jakov, Jakovian, Jakub, Jakubek, Jekebs

Jamaal (Arabic) an alternate form of Jamal.

Jamal (Arabic) handsome.
Jahmal, Jahmall, Jahmalle, Jahmel, Jahmil, Jahmile, Jam, Jamaal, Jamael, Jamahl, Jamail, Jamala, Jamale, Jamall, Jamar, Jamel, Jamil, Jammal, Jarmal, Jaumal, Jemal, Jermal

Jamar (American) a form of Jamal.

Jamar *(cont.)*
**Jam, Jamaar, Jamaari,
Jamahrae, Jamara, Jamarl,
Jamarr, Jamarvis, Jamaur,
Jarmar, Jarmarr, Jaumar,
Jemaar, Jemar, Jimar**

Jamel (Arabic) an alternate
form of Jamal.
**Jameel, Jamele, Jamell,
Jamelle, Jammel, Jarmel,
Jaumell, Je-Mell, Jimell**

James (Hebrew) supplanter,
substitute. (English) a form
of Jacob. Bible: James the
Great and James the Lesser
were two of the Twelve
Apostles. See also Diego,
Santiago, Seamus.
**Jacques, Jago, Jaime,
Jaimes, Jakome, Jamesie,
Jamesy, Jamie, Jas, Jasha,
Jay, Jaymes, Jem, Jemes,
Jim**

Jameson (English) son
of James.
**Jamerson, Jamesian,
Jamison, Jaymeson**

Jamie (English) a familiar
form of James.
**Jaime, Jaimey, Jaimie,
Jame, Jamee, Jamey,
Jameyel, Jami, Jamian,
Jammie, Jammy, Jayme,
Jaymee, Jaymie**

Jamil (Arabic) an alternate
form of Jamal.
**Jamiel, Jamiell, Jamielle,
Jamile, Jamill, Jamille,
Jamyl, Jarmil**

Jamison (English) son of
James.
**Jamiesen, Jamieson,
Jamisen**

Jan (Dutch, Slavic) a form
of John.
**Jaan, Janne, Jano, Janson,
Jenda, Yan**

Jared (Hebrew)
descendant.
**Jahred, Jaired, Jarad,
Jareid, Jarid, Jarod, Jarred,
Jarrett, Jarrod, Jarryd,
Jerad, Jered, Jerod, Jerrad,
Jerred, Jerrod, Jerryd,
Jordan**

Jarell (Scandinavian)
a form of Gerald.
**Jairell, Jareil, Jarel, Jarelle,
Jarrell, Jarryl, Jayryl, Jerel,
Jerell, Jerrell, Jharell**

Jaron (Hebrew) he will
sing; he will cry out.
**Jaaron, Jairon, Jaren,
Jarone, Jayron, Jayronn,
Je Ronn, J'ron**

Jarred (Hebrew) an alter-
nate form of Jared.
**Ja'red, Jarrad, Jarrayd,
Jarrid, Jarrod, Jarryd,
Jerrid**

Jarrell (English) a form
of Gerald.
**Jarel, Jarell, Jarrel, Jerall,
Jerel, Jerell**

Jarrett (English) a form
of Garrett, Jared.
**Jairett, Jaret, Jareth,
Jarett, Jaretté, Jarhett,**

Jarratt, Jarret, Jarrette, Jarrot, Jarrott, Jerrett

Jarrod (Hebrew) an alternate form of Jared.
Jarod, Jerod

Jarryd (Hebrew) an alternate form of Jared.
Jarrayd, Jaryd

Jarvis (German) skilled with a spear.
Jaravis, Jarv, Jarvaris, Jarvas, Jarvaska, Jarvey, Jarvie, Jarvorice, Jarvoris, Jarvous, Javaris, Jervey, Jervis

Jason (Greek) healer. Mythology: the hero who led the Argonauts in search of the Golden Fleece.
Jacen, Jaeson, Jahson, Jaisen, Jaison, Jasan, Jase, Jasen, Jasin, Jasten, Jasun, Jay, Jayson

Jaspal (Punjabi) living a virtuous lifestyle.

Jasper (French) green ornamental stone.
Jaspar, Jazper, Jespar, Jesper

Javan (Hebrew) Bible: son of Japheth.
Jaavon, Jahvaughan, Jahvine, Jahvon, JaVaughn, Javen, Javin, Javine, Javion, Javoanta, Javon, Javona, Javone, Javoney, Javoni, Javonn, Jayvin, Jayvion, Jayvon, Jevan

Javaris (English) a form of Jarvis.
Javaor, Javar, Javares, Javario, Javarius, Javaro, Javaron, Javarous, Javarre, Javarrious, Javarro, Javarte, Javarus, Javoris, Javouris

Javier (Spanish) owner of a new house. See also Xavier.
Jabier

Javon (Hebrew) an alternate form of Javan.

Jay (French) blue jay. (English) a short form of James, Jason.
Jae, Jai, Jave, Jaye, Jeays, Jeyes

Jayce (American) a combination of the initials J. + C.
JC, J.C., Jaycee, Jay Cee

Jayme (English) an alternate form of Jamie.
Jaymes, Jayms

Jaymes (English) an alternate form of James.
Jayms

Jayson (Greek) an alternate form of Jason.
Jaycent, Jaysen, Jaysin, Jayssen, Jaysson

Jean (French) a form of John.
Jéan, Jean-Francois, Jean-Michel, Jeannah, Jeannie, Jeannot, Jeanot, Jean-Philippe, Jeanty, Jene

Jed (Hebrew) a short form
of Jedidiah. (Arabic) hand.
Jedd, Jeddy, Jedi

Jedidiah (Hebrew) friend
of God, beloved of God.
**Jebediah, Jed, Jedediah,
Jedediha, Jedidia,
Jedidiah, Yedidya**

Jeff (English) a short form
of Jefferson, Jeffrey.
A familiar form of Geoffrey.
**Jefe, Jeffe, Jeffey, Jeffie,
Jeffy, Jhef**

Jefferson (English) son
of Jeff. History: Thomas
Jefferson was the third
U.S. president.
Jeferson, Jeff, Jeffers

Jeffery (English) an alter-
nate form of Jeffrey.
**Jefery, Jeffeory, Jefferay,
Jeffereoy, Jefferey,
Jefferie, Jeffory**

Jeffrey (English) divinely
peaceful. See also
Geoffrey.
**Jeff, Jefferies, Jeffery,
Jeffree, Jeffrery, Jeffrie,
Jeffries, Jeffry, Jefre, Jefry,
Jeoffroi, Joffre, Joffrey**

Jeffry (English) an alternate
form of Jeffrey.

Jerad, Jered (Hebrew)
alternate forms of Jared.
Jeread, Jeredd

Jerald (English) a form
of Gerald.

**Jeraldo, Jerold, Jerral,
Jerrald, Jerrold, Jerry**

Jeramie, Jeramy (Hebrew)
alternate forms of Jeremy.
**Jerame, Jeramee, Jeramey,
Jerami, Jerammie**

Jerel, Jerell (English) forms
of Jarell.
**Jerelle, Jeril, Jerrail, Jerral,
Jerrall, Jerrel, Jerrill,
Jerrol, Jerroll, Jerryll, Jeryl**

Jereme, Jeremey
(Hebrew) alternate forms
of Jeremy.
Jarame

Jeremiah (Hebrew) God
will uplift. Bible: a great
Hebrew prophet.
**Geremiah, Jaramia,
Jem, Jemeriah, Jemiah,
Jeramiah, Jeramiha,
Jere, Jereias, Jeremaya,
Jeremi, Jeremia, Jeremial,
Jeremias, Jeremija,
Jeremy, Jerimiah,
Jerimiha, Jerimya,
Jermiah, Jermija, Jerry**

Jeremie, Jérémie
(Hebrew) alternate forms
of Jeremy.
Jeremi, Jérémie, Jeremii

Jeremy (English) a form
of Jeremiah.
**Jaremay, Jaremi, Jaremy,
Jem, Jemmy, Jerahmy,
Jeramie, Jeramy, Jere,
Jereamy, Jereme, Jeremee,
Jeremey, Jeremie, Jérémie,
Jeremry, Jérémy, Jeremye,**

**Jereomy, Jeriemy, Jerime,
Jerimy, Jermey, Jeromy,
Jerremy**

Jermaine (English) sprout,
bud.
**Jarman, Jeremaine,
Jeremane, Jerimane,
Jermain, Jermane,
Jermanie, Jermayn,
Jermayne, Jermiane,
Jermine, Jer-Mon,
Jhirmaine**

Jermey (English) an alter-
nate form of Jeremy.
**Jerme, Jermee, Jermere,
Jermery, Jermie, Jhermie**

Jerome (Latin) holy.
**Gerome, Jere, Jeroen,
Jerom, Jérome, Jérôme,
Jeromo, Jeromy, Jeron,
Jerónimo, Jerrome,
Jerromy**

Jeromy (Latin) an alternate
form of Jerome.
Jeromey, Jeromie

Jeron (English) a form
of Jerome.
**Jéron, Jerone, Jeronimo,
Jerron, J'ron**

Jerrard (French) a form
of Gerard.
**Jarard, Jarrard, Jerard,
Jerardo, Jeraude**

Jerrod, Jerod (Hebrew)
alternate forms of Jarrod.

Jerry (German) mighty
spearman. (English) a

familiar form of Gerald,
Gerard. See also Gerry.
**Jehri, Jere, Jeree, Jeris,
Jerison, Jerri, Jerrie**

Jess (Hebrew) a short form
of Jesse.

Jesse (Hebrew) wealthy.
Bible: the father of David.
**Jescey, Jesee, Jesi, Jesie,
Jess, Jessé, Jessee, Jessey,
Jessi, Jessie, Jessy**

Jessie (Hebrew) an alternate form of Jesse.

Jesus (Hebrew) God is my
salvation. An alternate
form of Joshua. Bible: son
of Mary and Joseph,
believed by Christians to
be the Son of God. See
also Joshua.
Jecho, Jesús, Josu

Jim (Hebrew) supplanter,
substitute. (English)
a short form of James.
Jimbo, Jimi, Jimmy

Jimmie (English) an alternate form of Jimmy.
Jimmee

Jimmy (English) a familiar
form of Jim.
**Jimmey, Jimmie, Jimmyjo,
Jimy**

Joachim (Hebrew) God will
establish. See also Akeem.
**Joakim, Joaquim, Joaquín,
Jov**

Joaquin (Spanish) a form of Joachim.
Jehoichin, Joaquin, Jocquin, Jocquinn, Juaquin

Jody (Hebrew) a familiar form of Joseph.
Jodey, Jodi, Jodie, Jodiha, Joedy

Joe (Hebrew) a short form of Joseph.
Jo, Joely, Joey

Joel (Hebrew) God is willing. Bible: an Old Testament Hebrew prophet.
Jôel, Joël, Joell, Joelle, Joely, Jole, Yoel

Joey (Hebrew) a familiar form of Joe, Joseph.

John (Hebrew) God is gracious. Bible: name honoring John the Baptist and John the Evangelist. See also Evan, Giovanni, Hans, Ian, Ivan, Sean, Zane.
Jack, Jacsi, Jaenda, Jahn, Jan, Janak, Janco, Janek, Janis, Janne, János, Jansen, Jantje, Jantzen, Jas, Jean, Jehan, Jen, Jenkin, Jenkyn, Jens, Jhan, Jhanick, Jhon, Jian, Joáo, João, Jock, Joen, Johan, Johann, Johne, Johnl, Johnlee, Johnnie, Johnny, Johnson, Jon, Jonam, Jonas, Jone, Jones, Jonté, Jovan, Juan, Juhana

Johnathan (Hebrew) an alternate form of Jonathan.
Jhonathan, Johathe, Johnatan, Johnathaon, Johnathen, Johnatten, Johniathin, Johnothan, Johnthan

Johnathon (Hebrew) an alternate form of Jonathon.

Johnnie (Hebrew) a familiar form of John.
Johnie, Johnier, Johnni, Johnsie, Jonni, Jonnie

Johnny (Hebrew) a familiar form of John.
Jantje, Jhonny, Johney, Johnney, Johny, Jonny

Johnson (English) son of John.
Johnston, Jonson

Jon (Hebrew) an alternate form of John. A short form of Jonathan.
J'on, Joni, Jonn, Jonnie, Jonny, Jony

Jonah (Hebrew) dove. Bible: an Old Testament prophet who was swallowed by a large fish.
Giona, Jona, Yonah

Jonas (Lithuanian) a form of John. (Hebrew) he accomplishes.
Jonelis, Jonukas, Jonus, Jonutis, Joonas

Jonathan (Hebrew) gift of God. Bible: the son

of King Saul who became a loyal friend of David.
Janathan, Johnathan, Jon, Jonatan, Jonatane, Jonate, Jonatha, Jonathen, Jonathon, Jonattan, Jonethen, Jonnatha, Jonnathan, Jonnattan, Jonothan

Jonathon (Hebrew) an alternate form of Jonathan.
Joanathon, Johnathon, Jonothon, Jounathon, Yanaton

Jordan (Hebrew) descending.
Jared, Jordaan, Jordae, Jordain, Jordaine, Jordany, Jordáo, Jorden, Jordenn, Jordi, Jordie, Jordin, Jordon, Jordy, Jordyn, Jori, Jorrdan, Jory, Jourdain, Jourdan

Jordon (Hebrew) an alternate form of Jordan.
Jeordon, Johordan

Jordy (Hebrew) a familiar form of Jordan.

Jorge (Spanish) a form of George.
Jorrín

Jory (Hebrew) a familiar form of Jordan.
Joar, Joary, Jori, Jorie

Jose (Spanish) a form of Joseph.
Josean, Josecito, Josee, Joseito, Joselito, Josey

Josef (German, Portuguese, Czech, Scandinavian) a form of Joseph.
Joosef, Joseff, Josif, Jozef, József, Juzef

Joseph (Hebrew) God will add, God will increase. Bible: in the Old Testament, the son of Jesse who came to rule Egypt; in the New Testament, the husband of Mary. See also Giuseppe, Yusuf.
Jazeps, Jo, Jobo, Jody, Joe, Joeseph, Joey, Jojo, Joop, Joos, Jooseppi, Jopie, José, Joseba, Josef, Josep, Josephat, Josephe, Josephie, Josephus, Josheph, Josip, Jóska, Joza, Joze, Jozef, Jozhe, Jozio, Jozka, Jozsi, Jozzepi, Jupp, Juziu

Josh (Hebrew) a short form of Joshua.
Joshe

Joshua (Hebrew) God is my salvation. Bible: led the Israelites into the Promised Land. See also Jesus.
Johsua, Johusa, Josh, Joshau, Joshaua, Joshauh, Joshawa, Joshawah, Joshia, Joshu, Joshuaa, Joshuah, Joshuea, Joshula, Joshus, Joshusa, Joshuwa, Joshwa, Josue, Jousha, Jozshua, Jozsua, Jozua, Jushua

Josiah (Hebrew) fire of the Lord.
Joshiah, Josia, Josiahs, Josian, Josias, Josie

Josue (Hebrew) an alternate form of Joshua.
Joshue, Josu, Josua, Josuha, Jozus

Jovan (Latin) Jove-like, majestic. (Slavic) a form of John. Mythology: Jove, also known as Jupiter, was the supreme Roman god.
Jovaan, Jovani, Jovanic, Jovann, Jovanni, Jovannie, Jovannis, Jovanny, Jovany, Jovenal, Jovenel, Jovi, Jovian, Jovin, Jovito, Jovoan, Jovon, Jovonn, Jovonne, Yovan

Jr (Latin) a short form of Junior.
Jr.

Juan (Spanish) a form of John.
Juanch, Juanchito, Juanito, Juann, Juaun

Judd (Hebrew) praised.
Jud, Judson

Jude (Latin) a form of Judd. Bible: one of the Christian apostles, author of the New Testament book, "The Epistle of Saint Jude."

Judson (English) son of Judd.

Julian (Greek, Latin) an alternate form of Julius.
Jolyon, Juliaan, Juliano, Julien, Jullian, Julyan

Julien (Latin) an alternate form of Julian.

Julio (Hispanic) a form of Julius.

Julius (Greek, Latin) youthful, downy bearded. History: Julius Caesar was a great Roman emperor.
Jolyon, Julas, Jule, Jules, Julen, Jules, Julian, Julias, Julie, Julio, Juliusz

Junior (Latin) young.
Jr, Junious, Junius

Justin (Latin) just, righteous.
Jestin, Jobst, Joost, Jost, Jusa, Just, Justain, Justan, Justas, Justek, Justen, Justice, Justinas, Justine, Justinian, Justinius, Justinn, Justino, Justins, Justinus, Justo, Juston, Justton, Justun, Justyn

Justyn (Latin) an alternate form of Justin.
Justn

K

Kacey (Irish) an alternate form of Casey. (American) a combination of the initials K. + C.
Kace, Kacee, Kacy, Kaesy, Kase, Kasey, Kasie, Kasy, Kaycee

Kade (Scottish) wetlands. (American) a combination of the initials K. + D.
Kadee, Kaydee

Kai (Welsh) keeper of the keys. (Hawaiian) sea.

Kale (Hawaiian) a familiar form of Carl.
Kalee, Kaleu, Kaley, Kali, Kalin, Kayle

Kaleb (Hebrew) an alternate form of Caleb.
Kal, Kalab, Kalb, Kale, Kalev, Kalib, Kilab

Kalen, Kalin (Arabic) alternate forms of Kale. (Irish) alternate forms of Kellen.

Kalvin (Latin) an alternate form of Calvin.
Kal, Kalv, Vinny

Kameron (Scottish) an alternate form of Cameron.
Kam, Kamey, Kammy, Kamran, Kamren, Kamron

Kane (Welsh) beautiful. (Irish) tribute. (Japanese) golden. (Hawaiian) eastern sky.
Kahan, Kain, Kainan, Kaine, Kainen, Kaney, Kayne

Kareem (Arabic) noble; distinguished.
Karee, Karem, Kareme, Karim, Karriem

Karim (Arabic) an alternate form of Kareem.

Karl (German) an alternate form of Carl.
Kaarle, Kaarlo, Kale, Kalle, Kalman, Kálmán, Karcsi, Karel, Kari, Karlen, Karlitis, Karlo, Karlos, Karlton, Karlus, Karol, Kjell

Kasey (Irish) an alternate form of Casey.

Kayle (Hebrew) faithful dog.

Keaton (English) where hawks fly.
Keaten, Keeton, Keetun

Keegan (Irish) little; fiery.
Kaegan, Keagen, Kegan, Keghan, Kegun

Keenan (Irish) little Keene.
Keanan, Keanen, Keannan, Keenen, Keenon, Kenan, Keynan, Kienan, Kienen, Kienon

Keith (Welsh) forest.
(Scottish) battle place.
**Keath, Keeth, Keithen,
Keithon**

Kellen (Irish) mighty
warrior.
**Kaelan, Kailen, Kalan,
Kalen, Kalin, Kallen,
Kaylen, Keelan, Keilan,
Keillan, Kelden, Kellan,
Kelle, Kellin, Kelynn**

Kelly (Irish) warrior.
**Kelle, Kellen, Kelley, Kelli,
Kely**

Kelsey (Scandinavian)
island of ships.
**Kelcy, Kelse, Kelsie, Kelsy,
Kesley, Kesly**

Kelvin (Irish, English)
narrow river. Geography:
a river in Scotland.
**Kelvan, Kelven, Kelvyn,
Kelwin, Kelwyn**

Ken (Japanese) one's own
kind. (Scottish) a short
form of Kendall, Kendrick,
Kenneth.
Kena, Kenn, Keno

Kendall (English) valley
of the river Kent.
**Ken, Kendal, Kendale,
Kendali, Kendel, Kendell,
Kendrall, Kendrell,
Kendryll**

Kendrick (Irish) son of
Henry. (Scottish) royal
chieftain.
**Ken, Kendric, Kendricks,
Kendrik, Kendrix,**

**Kendryck, Keondric,
Keondrick**

Kenneth (Irish) handsome.
(English) royal oath.
**Ken, Keneth, Kennet,
Kennethen, Kennett,
Kennieth, Kennith,
Kennth, Kenny, Kennyth**

Kenny (Scottish) a familiar
form of Kenneth.
**Keni, Kenney, Kennie,
Kinnie**

Kent (Welsh) white; bright.
(English) a short form of
Kenton. Geography:
a county in England.

Kenton (English) from
Kent, England.
**Kent, Kenten, Kentin,
Kentonn**

Kentrell (English) king's
estate.

Keon (Irish) a form of Evan.
**Keeon, Keion, Keionne,
Keondre, Keone, Keontae,
Keontrye, Keony, Keyon,
Kian, Kion**

Kerry (Irish) dark,
dark haired.
**Keary, Keri, Kerrey, Kerri,
Kerrie**

Kevan (Irish) an alternate
form of Kevin.
Kavan

Keven (Irish) an alternate
form of Kevin.
Keve

Kevin (Irish) handsome.
Keevin, Keevon, Kev, Kevan, Keven, Keveon, Keverne, Kévin, Kevinn, Kevins, Kevion, Kevis, Kevn, Kevon, Kevron, Kevvy, Kevyn

Khalid (Arabic) eternal.
Khaled

Khalil (Arabic) friend.
Kahlil, Kaleel, Kalil, Khalee, Khali, Khalial, Khaliyl

Kiel (Irish) an alternate form of Kyle.

Kieran (Irish) little and dark; little Keir.
Keiran, Keiren, Keiron, Kern, Kernan, Kiernan, Kieron, Kyran

Kim (Greek) hollow vessel. (English) warrior chief.
Kimie, Kimmy

Kirby (Scandinavian) church village. (English) cottage by the water.
Kerbey, Kerbie, Kerby, Kirbey, Kirbie, Kirkby

Kirk (Scandinavian) church.
Kerk

Kody (English) an alternate form of Cody.
Kodey, Kodi, Kodie, Koty

Kolby (English) an alternate form of Colby.
Kelby, Kole, Kollby

Konrad (German) a form of Conrad.
Khonrad, Koen, Koenraad, Kon, Konn, Konney, Konni, Konnie, Konny, Konrád, Konrade, Konrado, Kord, Kort, Kunz

Korey (Irish) an alternate form of Corey, Kory.
Kore, Korio, Korria, Korrye

Kory (Irish) an alternate form of Corey.
Korey, Kori, Korie, Korrey, Korrie, Korry

Kraig (Irish, Scottish) an alternate form of Craig.
Kraggie, Kraggy

Kris (Greek) an alternate form of Chris. A short form of Kristian, Kristofer, Kristopher.
Kriss, Krys

Kristian (Greek) an alternate form of Christian.
Kerstan, Khristos, Kit, Kris, Krischan, Krist, Kristar, Kristek, Krister, Kristjan, Kristo, Kristos, Krists, Krystek, Krystian, Khrystiyan

Kristofer (Swedish) a form of Kristopher.
Kristef, Kristoffer, Kristofor, Kristus

Kristoph (French) a form
of Kristopher.
Kristophe

Kristopher (Greek) Christ-
bearer. An alternate form
of Christopher.
**Kit, Kris, Kristfer, Kristfor,
Kristo, Kristóf, Kristofer,
Kristoforo, Kristoph,
Kristophor, Kristos,
Krists, Krzysztof**

Kurt (Latin, German,
French) courteous;
enclosure. A short form
of Kurtis. An alternate
form of Curt.
Kort, Kuno

Kurtis (Latin, French) an
alternate form of Curtis.
Kurt, Kurtice, Kurtiss

Kyele (Irish) an alternate
form of Kyle.

Kyle (Irish) narrow piece
of land; place where cattle
graze. (Yiddish) crowned
with laurels.
**Kiel, Kilan, Kile, Kilen,
Kiley, Ky, Kye, Kyele,
Kylan, Kylen, Kyler, Kylie,
Kyrell**

Kyler (English) a form
of Kyle.

L

Lamar (German) famous
throughout the land.
(French) sea, ocean.
**Lamair, Lamario, Lamaris,
Lamarr, Lamarre, Larmar,
Lemar**

Lamont (Scandinavian)
lawyer.
**Lamaunt, Lamonte,
Lamontie, Lemont**

Lance (Latin) light spear.
(German) land.
Lancy, Lantz, Lanz, Launce

Landen (English) an alternate form of Landon.

Landon (English) open,
grassy meadow.
Landan, Landen, Landin

Lane (English) narrow road.
Laney, Lanie, Layne

Lanny (American) a familiar
form of Laurence,
Lawrence.
Lannie, Lennie

Laron (French) thief.
**Laran, La'ron, La Ron,
Laronn, La Ruan**

Larry (Latin) a familiar
form of Lawrence.
Larrie, Lary

Lars (Scandinavian) a form
of Lawrence.
Laris, Larris, Larse, Larsen,
Larson, Larsson, Lasse,
Laurans, Laurits, Lavrans,
Lorens

Laurence (Latin) crowned
with laurel. An alternate
form of Lawrence.
Lanny, Lauran, Laurance,
Laureano, Lauren,
Laurencho, Laurencio,
Laurens, Laurent,
Laurentij, Laurentios,
Laurentiu, Laurentius,
Laurentzi, Laurenz,
Laurie, Laurin, Lauris,
Laurits, Lauritz, Laurnet,
Lauro, Laurus, Lavrenti,
Lurance

Lawrence (Latin) crowned
with laurel.
Labrentsis, Laiurenty,
Lanny, Lanty, Larance,
Laren, Larian, Larien,
Laris, Larka, Larrance,
Larrence, Larry, Lars,
Larya, Laurence, Lavrenti,
Law, Lawerance,
Lawrance, Lawren,
Lawrey, Lawrie, Lawron,
Lawry, Lencho, Lon,
Lóránt, Loreca, Loren,
Loretto, Lorenzo, Lorne,
Lourenco, Lowrance

Layne (English) an alternate
form of Lane.

Lazaro (Hebrew) God has
helped.

Lazarillo, Lazarito,
Lazzaro

Lee (English) a short form
of Farley and names
containing "lee."
Leigh

Leif (Scandinavian)
beloved.
Laif, Lief

Leigh (English) an alternate
form of Lee.

Leland (English) meadow-
land; protected land.
Lealand, Lee, Leeland,
Leigh, Leighland, Lelan,
Lelann, Leyland

Leo (Latin) lion.
Lavi, Leão, Lee, Leib,
Leibel, Leos, Leosko, Léo,
Léocadie, Leos, Leosoko,
Lev, Lio, Lion, Liutas,
Lyon, Nardek

Leon (Greek, German)
a short form of Leonard.
Leo, Léon, Leonas, Léonce,
Leoncio, Leondris, Leone,
Leonek, Leonetti, Leoni,
Leonid, Leonidas,
Leonirez, Leonizio,
Leonon, Leons, Leontes,
Leontios, Leontrae, Liutas

Leonard (German) brave
as a lion.
Leanard, Lee, Len, Lena,
Lenard, Lennard, Lennart,
Lenny, Leno, Leon,
Leonaldo, Léonard,
Leonardis, Leonardo,

Leonard (cont.)
Leonart, Leonerd,
Leonhard, Leonidas,
Leontes, Lernard, Lienard,
Linek, Lnard, Lon,
Londard, Lonnard, Lonya,
Lynnard

Leonardo (Italian) a form
of Leonard.

Leonel (English) little lion.
See also Lionel.

Leroy (French) king.
Lee, Leeroy, LeeRoy, Leigh,
Lerai, Leroi, LeRoi, LeRoy,
Roy

Leslie (Scottish) gray
fortress.
Lee, Leigh, Les, Leslea,
Leslee, Lesley, Lesly,
Lezlie, Lezly

Lester (Latin) chosen
camp. (English) from
Leicester, England.
Leicester, Les

Levi (Hebrew) joined in
harmony. Bible: the son
of Jacob; the priestly tribe
of Israel.
Leavi, Leevi, Lev, Levey,
Levie, Levin, Levitis, Levy,
Lewi

Lewis (English) a form of
Louis.
Lew, Lewes, Lewie, Lewy

Liam (Irish) a form of
William.

Lincoln (English) settlement by the pool. History:
Abraham Lincoln was the
sixteenth U.S. president.
Linc, Lincon

Lindsay (English) an alternate form of Lindsey.
Linsay

Lindsey (English) linden-
tree island.
Lind, Lindsay, Lindsee,
Lindsy, Linsey, Lyndsay,
Lyndsey, Lyndsie, Lynzie

Lionel (French) lion cub.
See also Leonel.
Lional, Lionell, Lionello,
Lynel, Lynell, Lyonel

Lloyd (Welsh) gray haired;
holy. See also Floyd.
Loy, Loyd, Loyde, Loydie

Logan (Irish) meadow.
Logen

Lonnie (German, Spanish)
a familiar form of Alonzo.
Lonnell, Lonniel, Lonny

Loren (Latin) a short form
of Lawrence.
Lorin, Lorren, Lorrin,
Loryn

Lorenzo (Italian, Spanish)
a form of Lawrence.
Larinzo, Lerenzo, Lorenc,
Lorence, Lorenco,
Lorencz, Lorens, Lorentz,
Lorenz, Lorenza, Loretto,
Lorinc, Lörinc, Lorinzo,
Loritz, Lorrenzo, Lorrie,
Lorry, Renzo, Zo

Lorne (Latin) a short form of Lawrence.
Lorn, Lornie

Louis (German) famous warrior. See also Luigi.
Lash, Lashi, Lasho, Lewis, Lou, Loudovicus, Louie, Lucho, Lude, Ludek, Ludirk, Ludis, Ludko, Ludwig, Lughaidh, Lui, Luigi, Luis, Luki, Lutek

Lowell (French) young wolf. (English) beloved.
Lovell, Lowe, Lowel

Luc (French) a form of Luke.
Luce

Lucas (German, Irish, Danish, Dutch) light; bringer of light.
Luca, Lucassie, Luckas, Lucus

Luigi (Italian) a form of Louis.
Lui, Luigino

Luis (Spanish) a form of Louis.
Luise, Luiz

Lukas (Greek, Czech, Swedish) a form of Luke.
Loukas, Lukash, Lukasha, Lukass, Lukasz

Luke (Latin) a form of Lucius. Bible: author of the Gospel of Saint Luke and Acts of the Apostles—two New Testament books.
Luc, Luck, Lucky, Luk, Luka, Lúkács, Lukas, Luken, Lukes, Lukus, Lukyan, Lusio

Luther (German) famous warrior. History: the Protestant reformer Martin Luther was one of the central figures of the Reformation.
Lothar, Lutero, Luthor

Lyle (French) island.
Lisle, Ly, Lysle

Lyndon (English) linden-tree hill. History: Lyndon B. Johnson was the thirty-sixth U.S. president.
Lin, Lindon, Lyden, Lydon, Lyn, Lynden, Lynn

Lynn (English) waterfall; brook.
Lyn, Lynell, Lynette, Lynnard, Lynoll

M

Mack (Scottish) a short form of names beginning with "Mac" and "Mc."
Macke, Mackey, Mackie, Macklin, Macks

Mackenzie (Irish) son of the wise leader.

Mackenzie *(cont.)*
**Mackenxo, Mackenzey,
Mackenzi, MacKenzie,
Mackenzly, Mackenzy,
Mackienzie, Mackinsey,
Makenzie, McKenzie**

Madison (English) son
of Maude; good son.
**Maddie, Maddison,
Maddy, Madisson,
Son, Sonny**

Malachi (Hebrew) angel of
God. Bible: the last canon-
ical Hebrew prophet.
**Maeleachlainn, Mal,
Malachia, Malachie,
Malachy, Malchija,
Malechy, Málik**

Malcolm (Scottish)
follower of Saint Columba,
an early Scottish saint.
(Arabic) dove.
**Mal, Malcolum, Malcom,
Malcum, Malkolm**

Malik (Arabic) a form of
Malachi. (Punjabi) lord,
master.
**Maalik, Malak, Málik,
Malikh, Maliq, Malique,
Mallik**

Mandeep (Punjabi) mind
full of light.
Mandieep

Manuel (Hebrew) a short
form of Emmanuel.
**Maco, Mango, Mannuel,
Manny, Mano, Manolón,
Manual, Manue, Manuelli,**
**Manuelo, Manuil,
Manyuil, Minel**

Marc (French) a form
of Mark.
Marc-André, Mark-Andre

Marcel (French) a form
of Marcus.
Marcell, Marsale, Marsel

Marcello (Italian) a form
of Marcus.
**Marcelo, Marchello,
Marsello, Marselo**

Marco (Italian) a form of
Marcus. History: Marco
Polo was the thirteenth-
century Venetian traveler
who explored Asia.
Marcko, Marko

Marcos (Spanish) a form
of Marcus.
Markos, Markose

Marcus (Latin) martial,
warlike.
**Marc, Marcas, Marcellus,
Marcio, Marckus, Marco,
Marcos, Marcous, Marek,
Mark, Markov, Markus**

Mario (Italian) a form of
Marion.
Marios, Marrio

Marion (French) bitter; sea
of bitterness. A masculine
form of Mary.
Mariano

Mark (Latin) an alternate
form of Marcus. Bible:
author of the New

Testament book, the
*Gospel According to
Saint Mark.*
**Marc, Marek, Marian,
Mariano, Marke, Markee,
Markel, Markell, Markey,
Marko, Markos, Márkus,
Marque, Martial, Marx**

Marko (Latin) an alternate
form of Marco, Mark.
Markco

Markus (Latin) an alternate
form of Marcus.
**Markas, Markcus,
Markcuss, Marqus**

Marlin (English) deep-sea
fish.
Marlion

Marlon (French) a form
of Merlin.

Marques (Portuguese)
nobleman.
**Markes, Markques,
Marquest, Markqueus,
Marquez, Marqus**

Marquis (French)
nobleman.
**Marcquis, Marcuis,
Markis, Markuis,
Marquee, Marqui,
Marquie, Marquise,
Marquist**

Marshall (French)
caretaker of the horses;
military title.
**Marschal, Marsh, Marshal,
Marshel, Marshell**

Martell (English)
hammerer.
Martel

Martin (Latin) martial,
warlike. History: Martin
Luther King, Jr. led the
civic rights movement and
won the Nobel Peace
Prize.
**Maartin, Mairtin,
Marciano, Marcin,
Marinos, Marius, Mart,
Martan, Marten, Martijn,
Martinas, Martine,
Martinez, Martinho,
Martiniano, Martinien,
Martino, Martins, Marto,
Marton, Márton, Marts,
Marty, Martyn, Mattin,
Mertin, Morten, Moss**

Marty (Latin) a familiar
form of Martin.
Martey, Marti, Martie

Marvin (English) lover
of the sea.
**Marv, Marvein, Marven,
Marwin, Marwynn,
Mervin**

Mason (French) stone
worker.
Mace, Maison, Sonny

Massimo (Italian) greatest.
Massimiliano

Mathew (Hebrew) an alternate form of Matthew.

Mathieu (French) a form
of Matthew.

Mathieu (cont.)
Mathie, Mathieux,
Mathiew, Matthieu,
Matthiew, Mattieu,
Mattieux

Matt (Hebrew) a short
form of Matthew.
Mat

Matthew (Hebrew) gift
of God. Bible: author of
the New Testament book,
the Gospel According to
Saint Matthew.
Mads, Makaio, Maitiú,
Mata, Matai, Matek,
Mateo, Mateusz, Matfei,
Mathe, Matheson,
Matheu, Mathew,
Mathian, Mathias,
Mathieson, Mathieu,
Matro, Mats, Matt,
Matteus, Matthaeus,
Matthaios, Matthaus,
Matthäus, Mattheus,
Matthews, Mattmias,
Matty, Matvey, Matyas,
Mayhew

Maurice (Latin) dark
skinned; moor; marshland.
Mauli, Maur,
Maurance, Maureo,
Mauricio, Maurids,
Mauriece, Maurikas,
Maurin, Maurino,
Maurio, Maurise, Mauritz,
Maurius, Maurizio, Mauro,
Maurrel, Maurtel, Maury,
Maurycy, Meurig, Moore,
Morice, Moritz, Morrel,

Morrice, Morrie, Morrill,
Morris

Mauricio (Spanish) a form
of Maurice.

Max (Latin) a short form
of Maximilian, Maxwell.
Mac, Mack, Maks, Maxe,
Maxx, Maxy, Miksa

Maxime (French) most
excellent.
Maxim

Maximilian (Latin)
greatest.
Mac, Mack, Maixim,
Maksym, Massimiliano,
Max, Maxamillion,
Maxemilian, Maxemilion,
Maxi, Maximalian,
Maxime, Maximili,
Maximilia, Maximilianus,
Maximilien, Maximillian,
Maximillion, Máximo,
Maximos, Maxmilian,
Maxmillion, Maxon,
Maxymilian, Maxymillian,
Mayhew, Miksa

Maxwell (English) great
spring.
Max, Maxwel, Maxwill,
Maxy

Mckay (Scottish) son of the
rejoicing man.
Mackay, MacKay, McKay

Melvin (Irish) armored
chief. (English) mill friend;
council friend.

Malvin, Mel, Melvino,
Melvon, Melvyn, Melwin,
Melwyn, Melwynn

Merle (French) famous.
Meryl

Mervin (Irish) a form
of Marvin.
Merv, Mervyn, Mervynn,
Merwin, Merwinn,
Merwyn, Murvin, Murvyn,
Myrvyn, Myrvynn,
Myrwyn

Micah (Hebrew) an alter-
nate form of Michael.
Bible: a Hebrew prophet.
Mic, Micaiah, Michiah,
Mika, Mikah, Myca,
Mycah

Michael (Hebrew) who is
like God? See also Micah,
Miguel, Miles.
Machael, Machas, Mahail,
Maichail, Maikal, Makael,
Makal, Makel, Makell,
Makis, Meikel, Mekal,
Mekhail, Mhichael,
Micael, Micah, Micahel,
Mical, Micha, Michaele,
Michaell, Michail, Michak,
Michal, Michale, Michau,
Micheal, Micheil,
Michel, Michele, Michelet,
Michiel, Micho, Michoel,
Mick, Mickael, Mickey,
Mihail, Mihalje, Mihkel,
Mika, Mikael, Mikáele,
Mikal, Mike, Mikeal,
Mikel, Mikelis, Mikell,
Mikhail, Mikkel, Mikko,

Miksa, Milko, Miquel,
Mitchell, Mychael,
Mychajlo, Mychal, Mykal,
Mykhas

Micheal (Irish) a form
of Michael.

Michel (French) a form
of Michael.
Michaud, Miche, Michee,
Michon

Michele (Italian) a form
of Michael.

Mickey (Irish) a familiar
form of Michael.
Mick, Mickie, Micky, Miki,
Mique

Miguel (Portuguese,
Spanish) a form of
Michael.
Migeel, Migel, Miguelly,
Migui

Mikael (Swedish) a form
of Michael.
Mikaeel, Mikaele

Mikal (Hebrew) an alternate form of Michael.
Mekal

Mike (Hebrew) a short
form of Michael.
Mikey, Myk

Mikeal (Irish) a form
of Michael.

Mikel (Basque) a form
of Michael.
Mekel, Mekell, Mikell

Mikhail (Greek, Russian)
a form of Michael.

Mikhail *(cont.)*
Mekhail, Mihály, Mikhael, Mikhalis, Mikhial, Mikhos

Miles (Greek) millstone. (Latin) soldier. (German) merciful. (English) a short form of Michael.
Milas, Milles, Milo, Milson, Myles

Milton (English) mill town.
Milt, Miltie, Milty, Mylton

Mitch (English) a short form of Mitchell.

Mitchell (English) a form of Michael.
Mitch, Mitchael, Mitchall, Mitchel, Mitchele, Mitchelle, Mitchem, Mytch, Mytchell

Mohammad (Arabic) an alternate form of Mohammed.
Mahammad, Mohamad, Mohamid, Mohammadi, Mohammd, Mohammid, Mohanad, Mohmad

Mohammed (Arabic) praised. See also Ahmad.
Mahammed, Mahmúd, Mahomet, Mohamed, Mohamet, Mohammad, Mohaned, Mouhamed, Muhammad

Moises (Portuguese, Spanish) a form of Moses.
Moisés, Moisey, Moisis

Monte (Latin) mountain.
Montae, Montaé, Montay, Montee, Monti, Montoya, Monty

Montez (Spanish) dweller in the mountains.
Monteiz, Monteze, Montisze

Monty (English) a form of Monte.

Morgan (Scottish) sea warrior.
Morgen, Morgun, Morrgan

Morris (Latin) dark skinned; moor; marshland. (English) a form of Maurice.
Moris, Moriss, Morriss, Morry, Moss

Moses (Hebrew) drawn out of the water. (Egyptian) son, child. Bible: the Hebrew leader who brought the Ten Commandments down from Mount Sinai.
Moe, Moise, Moïse, Moisei, Moises, Moishe, Mose, Mosese, Mosiah, Mosie, Moss, Mosya, Mosze, Moszek, Mousa, Moyses, Moze

Moshe (Hebrew, Polish) an alternate form of Moses.
Mosheh

Muhammad (Arabic) an alternate form of

Mohammed. History:
the founder of the
Islamic religion.
**Muhamad, Muhamet,
Muhammadali,
Muhammed**

Murray (Scottish) sailor.
**Macmurray, Moray,
Murrey, Murry**

Mustafa (Arabic) chosen;
royal.
**Mostafa, Mostaffa,
Moustafa, Mustafah,
Mustapha**

Myles (Latin) soldier.
(German) an alternate
form of Miles.

Myron (Greek) fragrant
ointment.
**Mehran, Mehrayan, My,
Myran, Myrone, Ron**

N

Nathan (Hebrew) a short
form of Nathaniel. Bible:
an Old Testament prophet
who saved Solomon's
kingdom.
**Naethan, Nat, Nate,
Nathann, Nathean,
Nathen, Nathian, Nathin,
Nathon, Natthan,
Naythan**

Nathanael (Hebrew)
an alternate form of
Nathaniel.
Nathanae

Nathanial (Hebrew)
an alternate form of
Nathaniel.

Nathanie (Hebrew)
a familiar form of
Nathaniel.
Nathania, Nathanni

Nathaniel (Hebrew) gift
of God. Bible: one of the
Twelve Apostles.
**Nat, Natanael, Nataniel,
Nate, Nathan, Nathanael,
Nathanal, Nathaneal,
Nathaneil, Nathanel,
Nathaneol, Nathanial,
Nathanie, Nathanielle,
Nathanuel, Nathanyal,
Nathanyel, Natheal,
Nathel, Nathinel,
Nethaniel, Thaniel**

Nathen (Hebrew) an alternate form of Nathan.

Neal (Irish) an alternate
form of Neil.
**Neale, Neall, Nealle,
Nealon, Nealy**

Neil (Irish) champion.
**Neal, Neel, Neihl, Neile,
Neill, Neille, Nels, Nial,
Niall, Nialle, Niele, Niels,
Nigel, Nil, Niles, Nilo, Nils,
Nyle**

Nelson (English) son
of Neil.

Nelson (cont.)
Nealson, Neilson, Nellie,
Nels, Nelsen, Nilson,
Nilsson

Nevin (Irish) worshiper of
the saint. (English) middle;
herb.
Nefen, Nev, Nevan, Neven,
Nevins, Niven

Nicholas (Greek) victorious
people. Religion: the
patron saint of children.
See also Cole, Colin.
Niccolas, Nichalas,
Nichelas, Nichele, Nichlas,
Nichlos, Nichola, Nichole,
Nicholl, Nichols, Nick,
Nicklaus, Nickolas, Nicky,
Niclas, Niclasse, Nicolai,
Nicolas, Nicoles, Nicolis,
Nicoll, Nicolo, Nikhil,
Nikili, Nikita, Niklas,
Nikolas, Nikolos, Nils,
Nioclás, Niocol, Nycholas

Nick (English) a short form
of Dominic, Nicholas.
Nic, Nik

Nicklaus (Greek) an alter-
nate form of Nicholas.
Nicholaus, Nicklas,
Nickolau, Nickolaus,
Nicolaus, Niklaus,
Nikolaus

Nickolas (Greek) an alternate form of Nicholas.
Nickolaos, Nickolus

Nicola (Italian) a form
of Nicholas.
Nicol, Nicolao

Nicolas (Italian) a form
of Nicholas.
Nico, Nicolaas, Nicolás

Nigel (Latin) dark night.
Niegel, Nigal, Nigiel, Nigil,
Nigle, Nijel, Nye, Nygel

Nikolas (Greek) an alter-
nate form on Nicholas.
Nicanor, Nikalus, Nikola,
Nikolaas, Nikolao,
Nikolaos, Nikolis, Nikolos,
Nikos, Nilos, Nykolas

Noah (Hebrew) peaceful,
restful. Bible: the patriarch
who built the ark to sur-
vive the Great Flood.
Noach, Noak, Noe, Noé,
Noi

Noel (French) day of
Christ's birth.
Noel, Noél, Nole, Noli,
Nowel, Nowell

Nolan (Irish) famous;
noble.
Noland, Nolen, Nolin,
Nollan, Nolyn

Norman (French) norse-
man. History: a name for
the Scandinavians who
conquered Normandy
in the tenth century,
and who later conquered
England in 1066.
Norm, Normand, Normen,
Normie, Normy

O

Oliver (Latin) olive tree. (Scandinavian) kind; affectionate.
Nollie, Oilibhéar, Oliverio, Oliverios, Olivero, Olivier, Oliviero, Oliwa, Ollie, Olliver, Ollivor, Olvan

Olivier (French) a form of Oliver.

Omar (Arabic) highest; follower of the Prophet. (Hebrew) reverent.
Omair, Omari, Omarr, Omer, Umar

Oren (Hebrew) pine tree. (Irish) light skinned, white.
Oran, Orin, Oris, Orren, Orrin

Orlando (German) famous throughout the land. (Spanish) a form of Roland.
Lando, Olando, Olo, Orlan, Orland, Orlanda, Orlandus, Orlo, Orlondo, Orlondon

Orry (Latin) from the Orient.
Oarrie, Orrey, Orrie

Oscar (Scandinavian) divine spearman.
Oke, Oskar, Osker, Oszkar

Osvaldo (Spanish) a form of Oswald.
Osvald, Osvalda

Oswald (English) God's power; God's crest.
Osvaldo, Oswold, Ozzie

Otis (Greek) keen of hearing. (German) son of Otto.
Oates, Odis, Otes, Otess, Ottis, Otys

Otto (German) rich.
Odo, Otek, Otello, Otfried, Othello, Otho, Othon, Otik, Otilio, Otman, Oto, Otón, Otton, Ottone

Owen (Irish) born to nobility; young warrior. (Welsh) a form of Evan.
Owain, Owens, Owin, Uaine

P

Pablo (Spanish) a form of Paul.
Pable, Paublo

Paolo (Italian) a form of Paul.

Paris (Greek) lover.
Geography: the capital
of France. Mythology:
the prince of Troy who
started the Trojan War
by abducting Helen.
Paras, Paree, Parris

Parker (English) park
keeper.
Park

Pascal (French) born
on Easter or Passover.
**Pace, Pascale, Pascalle,
Paschal, Paschalis, Pascoe,
Pascow, Pascual, Pasquale**

Pasquale (Italian) a form
of Pascal.
Pascuale, Pasquel

Patrick (Latin) nobleman.
Religion: the patron saint
of Ireland.
**Paddy, Padraic, Pakelika,
Pat, Patek, Paton, Patric,
Patrice, Patricio, Patrik,
Patrique, Patrizius,
Patryck, Patryk, Pats,
Patsy**

Paul (Latin) small. Bible:
Saul, later renamed Paul,
was the first to bring
the teachings of Christ
to the Gentiles.
**Oalo, Paavo, Pablo, Pal,
Pál, Pall, Paolo, Pasha,
Pasko, Pauli, Paulia,
Paulin, Paulino, Paulis,
Paulo, Pauls, Paulus,
Pavel, Pavlos, Pawel, Pol**

Paulo (Portuguese,
Swedish, Hawaiian)
a form of Paul.

Payton (English) warrior's
town.
**Paiton, Pate, Payden,
Paydon, Peyton**

Pedro (Spanish) a form
of Peter.
Pedrin, Pedrín, Petronio

Percy (French) prisoner of
the valley.
**Pearcey, Pearcy, Percey,
Percie, Piercey, Piercy**

Perry (English) a familiar
form of Peter.
Parry, Perrie

Pete (English) a short
form of Peter.
**Peat, Peet, Petey, Peti,
Petie, Piet, Pit**

Peter (Greek, Latin) small
rock. Bible: Simon,
renamed Peter, was the
leader of the Twelve
Apostles.
**Panayiotos, Panos,
Peadair, Peder, Pedro,
Peers, Peeter, Peirce,
Pekelo, Per, Perico,
Perion, Perkin, Perren,
Perry, Petar, Pete, Péter,
Peteris, Peterke, Peterus,
Petr, Petras, Petros,
Petru, Petruno, Petter,
Peyo, Piaras, Pierce, Piero,
Pierre, Pieter, Pietrek,
Pietro, Piotr, Piter, Piti,
Pjeter, Pyotr**

Philip (Greek) lover of
horses. Bible: one of the
Twelve Apostles. See also
Felipe.
**Phelps, Phelipe, Phil,
Philipp, Philippe,
Philippo, Phillip, Phillipos,
Phillp, Philly, Philp, Piers,
Pilib, Pilipo, Pippo**

Philippe (French) a form
of Philip.
Philipe, Phillepe

Phillip (Greek) an alternate
form of Philip.
**Phil, Phillipos, Phillipp,
Phillips, Philly**

Pierce (English) a form
of Peter.
**Pearce, Pears, Pearson,
Pearsson, Peerce, Peers,
Peirce, Piercy, Piers,
Pierson, Piersson**

Pierre (French) a form
of Peter.
Peirre, Piere, Pierrot

Pierre-Luc (French) a combination of Pierre + Luc.

Pietro (Italian) a form
of Peter.

Preston (English) priest's
estate.
Prestin

Prince (Latin) chief; prince.
**Prence, Princeton, Prinz,
Prinze**

Q

Quentin (Latin) fifth.
(English) Queen's town.
**Qeuntin, Quantin, Quent,
Quenten, Quenton,
Quientin, Quienton,
Quintin, Quinton,
Qwentin**

Quincy (French) fifth son's
estate.
**Quincey, Quinn, Quinnsy,
Quinsey**

Quinn (Irish) a short form
of Quincy, Quinton.

Quintin (Latin) an alternate
form of Quentin.

Quinton (Latin) an alter-
nate form of Quentin.
**Quinn, Quinneton, Quint,
Quintan, Quintann,
Quinten, Quintin,
Quintus, Quitin, Quiton,
Qunton, Qwinton**

R

Rafael (Spanish) a form of Raphael.
Rafaelle, Rafaello, Rafaelo, Rafal, Rafeal, Rafeé, Rafel, Rafello, Raffael, Raffaelo, Raffeal

Raheem (Punjabi) compassionate God.

Rahim (Arabic) merciful.
Raheem, Raheim, Rahiem, Rahiim

Rahul (Arabic) traveler.

Ralph (English) wolf counselor.
Radolphus, Rafe, Ralf, Ralpheal, Ralphel, Ralphie, Ralston, Raoul, Raul, Rolf

Ramon (Spanish) a form of Raymond.
Ramon, Remone, Romone

Ramsey (English) ram's island.
Ram, Ramsay, Ramsy, Ramzee, Ramzi

Randal (English) an alternate form of Randall.
Randale, Randel, Randle

Randall (English) an alternate form of Randolph.
Randal, Randell, Randy

Randolph (English) shield-wolf.
Randall, Randol, Randolf, Randolfo, Randolpho, Randy, Ranolph

Randy (English) a familiar form of Rand, Randall, Randolph.
Randey, Randi, Randie, Ranndy

Raphael (Hebrew) God has healed. Bible: one of the archangels. Art: a prominent painter of the Italian Renaissance.
Rafael, Rafaele, Rafal, Raphaél, Raphale, Raphaello, Rapheal, Raphel, Raphello, Ray, Rephael

Rashad (Arabic) wise counselor.
Raashad, Rachad, Rachard, Rachaud, Raeshad, Raishard, Rashaad, Rashaud, Rashaude, Rashid, Rashod, Rashoda, Rashodd, Rayshod, Reshad, Rhashad, Rhashod, Rishad, Roshad

Rashawn (American) a combination of the prefix Ra + Shawn.

Rashann, Rashaun, Rashaw, Rashon, Rashun, Raushan, Raushawn, Rhashan, Rhashaun, Rhashawn

Rasheen (American) a combination of the prefix Ra + Sean.
Rashane, Rashean, Rashien, Rashiena

Raul (French) a form of Ralph.

Ravi (Hindi) sun. Religion: another name for the Hindu sun god Surya.
Ravee, Ravijot

Ray (French) kingly, royal. (English) a short form of Raymond.
Rae, Raye

Raymond (English) mighty; wise protector.
Radmond, Raemond, Raemondo, Raimondo, Raimundo, Ramón, Ramond, Ramonde, Ramone, Ray, Rayman, Raymand, Rayment, Raymon, Raymont, Raymund, Raymunde, Reamonn, Redmond

Raynard (French) wise; bold, courageous.

Reece (Welsh) enthusiastic; stream.
Reese, Reice, Rice

Reed (English) an alternate form of Reid.
Raeed, Read, Reyde

Reese (Welsh) an alternate form of Reece.
Rees, Reis, Rhys, Riess

Regan (Irish) little king.

Reggie (English) a familiar form of Reginald.

Reginal (English) a form of Reginald.

Reginald (English) king's advisor.
Reg, Reggie, Reggis, Reginal, Reginaldo, Reginale, Reginalt, Reginauld, Reginault, Reginel, Regnauld, Reinaldo, Ronald

Regis (Latin) regal.

Reid (English) redhead.
Read, Reed, Reide, Ried

Reinaldo (Spanish) a form of Reginald.

Remi, Rémi (French) from Rheims, France.
Remie, Remmie

Rene (French) reborn.
Renat, Renato, Renatus, Renault, Renee, Renny

Reuben (Hebrew) behold a son.
Reuban, Reubin, Reuven, Rheuben, Rube, Ruben, Rubey, Rubin, Ruby, Rueben

Rex (Latin) king.

Rhett (Welsh) an alternate form of Rhys. Literature: Rhett Butler was the hero

Rhett *(cont.)*
of Margaret Mitchell's
novel *Gone with the Wind.*

Rhys (Welsh) an alternate
form of Reece.
Rhett, Rice

Rian (Irish) little king.

Ricardo (Portuguese,
Spanish) a form of
Richard.
**Racardo, Recard, Ricaldo,
Ricard, Ricardos,
Riccardo, Ricciardo,
Richardo**

Richard (English) rich and
powerful ruler. See also
Aric.
**Reku, Ricardo, Rich,
Richar, Richards,
Richardson, Richart,
Richer, Richerd, Richie,
Richshard, Rick, Rickard,
Rickert, Rickey, Ricky,
Rico, Rihardos, Rihards,
Rikard, Riocard, Riócard,
Risa, Risardas, Rishard,
Ristéard, Ritchard, Rostik,
Rye, Rysio, Ryszard**

Rick (German) a short
form of Richard.
**Ric, Ricke, Rickey, Ricks,
Ricky, Rik, Riki, Rykk**

Rickey (English) a familiar
form of Richard, Rick.

Ricky (English) a familiar
form of Richard, Rick.
**Ricci, Rickey, Ricki, Rickie,
Riczi, Riki, Rikki, Rikky,
Riqui**

Rico (Spanish) a familiar
form of Richard.
Ric

Riley (Irish) valiant.
**Reilly, Rilley, Rilye, Rylee,
Ryley, Rylie**

Robbie (English) a familiar
form of Robert.
Robie, Robbi

Robby (English) a familiar
form of Robert.
Robbey, Robhy, Roby

Robert (English) famous
brilliance. See also Bob,
Bobby.
**Rab, Rabbie, Raby,
Riobard, Riobart, Rob,
Robars, Robart, Robbie,
Robby, Rober, Roberd,
Robers, Roberto, Roberts,
Robin, Robinson,
Roibeárd, Rosertas,
Rubert, Ruberto, Rudbert,
Rupert**

Roberto (Portuguese,
Spanish) a form of Robert.

Robin (English) a short
form of Robert.
**Robben, Robbin, Robbins,
Robbyn, Roben, Robinet,
Robinn, Robins, Robyn,
Roibín**

Rocco (Italian) rock.
**Rocca, Rocky, Roko,
Roque**

Rocky (American) a familiar
form of Rocco.
Rockey, Rockie

Roderick (German) famous ruler. See also Broderick.
Rhoderick, Rod, Rodderick, Roddrick, Roddy, Roderic, Roderich, Roderigo, Roderik, Roderyck, Rodgrick, Rodric, Rodrich, Rodrick, Rodricki, Rodrigo, Rodrigue, Rodrik, Rodrique, Rodrugue, Rodryck, Rodryk, Roodney, Rory, Rurik, Ruy

Rodger (German) an alternate form of Roger.
Rodge, Rodgy

Rodney (English) island clearing.
Rhodney, Rod, Rodnee, Rodni, Rodnie, Rodnne

Rodolfo (Spanish) a form of Rudolph.
Rodolpho, Rodulfo

Rodrick (German) an alternate form of Roderick.

Rodrigo (Italian, Spanish) a form of Roderick.

Roger (German) famous spearman.
Rodger, Rog, Rogelio, Rogerick, Rogerio, Rogers, Rogiero, Rojelio, Rüdiger, Ruggerio, Rutger

Roland (German) famous throughout the land. See also Orlando.
Loránd, Rawlins, Rolan, Rolanda, Rolando, Rolek,

Rolland, Rolle, Rollie, Rollin, Rollo, Rowe, Rowland, Ruland

Rolando (Portuguese, Spanish) a form of Roland.
Lando, Olo, Roldan, Roldán

Roman (Latin) from Rome, Italy.
Roma, Romain, Romanos, Romman, Romy

Ron (Hebrew) a short form of Aaron, Ronald.
Ronn

Ronald (Scottish) a form of Reginald.
Ranald, Ron, Ronal, Ronaldo, Ronney, Ronnie, Ronnold, Ronoldo

Ronnie (Scottish) a familiar form of Ronald.
Roni, Ronie, Ronney, Ronnie, Ronny

Roosevelt (Dutch) rose field. History: Theodore and Franklin D. Roosevelt were the twenty-sixth and thirty-second U.S. presidents, respectively.
Rosevelt

Rory (German) a familiar form of Roderick. (Irish) red king.
Rorey

Roscoe (Scandinavian) deer forest.
Rosco

Ross (Latin) rose. (Scottish)
peninsula. (French) red.
**Rosse, Rossell, Rossi,
Rossie, Rossy**

Roy (French) king. A short
form of Royce. See also
Leroy.
Rey, Roi, Ruy

Royce (English) son of Roy.
Roice, Roy

Ruben (Hebrew) an alternate form of Reuben.
Rube, Rubin, Ruby

Rudolph (German) famous
wolf.
**Raoul, Rezsó, Rodolfo,
Rodolph, Rodolphe,
Rolf, Ruda, Rudek,
Rudi, Rudolf, Rudolpho,
Rudolphus, Rudy**

Rudy (English) a familiar
form of Rudolph.
Ruddy, Ruddie, Rudey

Rufus (Latin) redhead.
**Rayfus, Rufe, Ruffis,
Ruffus, Rufino, Rufo,
Rufous**

Russell (French) redhead;
fox colored.
**Roussell, Rush, Russ,
Russel, Russelle, Rusty**

Rusty (French) a familiar
form of Russell.
Rustie, Rustin, Rustyn

Ryan (Irish) little king.
**Rhyan, Rhyne, Ryane,
Ryann, Ryen, Ryin, Ryne,
Ryon, Ryuan, Ryun**

Rylan (English) land where
rye is grown.
**Ryeland, Ryland, Rylin,
Rylund**

Ryne (Irish) an alternate
form of Ryan.

S

Salvador (Spanish) savior.
Salvadore

Salvatore (Italian) savior.
See also Xavier.
**Sal, Salbatore, Sallie,
Sally, Salvator, Salvidor,
Sauveur**

Sam (Hebrew) a short form
of Samuel.
**Samm, Sammy, Sem,
Shem, Shmuel**

Samír (Arabic) entertaining
companion.

Sammy (Hebrew) a familiar
form of Samuel.
**Saamy, Sameeh, Sameh,
Samey, Samie, Sammee,
Sammey, Sammie, Samy**

Samson (Hebrew) like the
sun. Bible: a strong man
betrayed by Delilah.
**Sampson, Sansao,
Sansom, Sansón, Shem,
Shimshon**

Samuel (Hebrew) heard God; asked of God. Bible: a famous Old Testament prophet and judge.
Sam, Samael, Samaru, Samauel, Samaul, Sambo, Sameul, Samiel, Sammail, Sammel, Sammuel, Sammy, Samo, Samouel, Samu, Samual, Samuele, Samuelis, Samuello, Samuil, Samuka, Samule, Samuru, Samvel, Sanko, Saumel, Schmuel, Shem, Shmuel, Simão, Simuel, Somhairle, Zamuel

Sandeep (Punjabi) enlightened.

Sandy (English) a familiar form of Alexander.
Sande, Sandey, Sandie

Santiago (Spanish) a form of James.

Sasha (Russian) a short form of Alexander.
Sacha, Sascha, Sausha

Saul (Hebrew) asked for, borrowed. Bible: in the Old Testament, a king of Israel and the father of Jonathan; in the New Testament, Saint Paul's original name was Saul.
Saül, Shaul, Sol, Solly

Schuyler (Dutch) sheltering.
Schuylar, Schylar, Schyler, Scoy, Scy, Skuyler, Sky, Skylar, Skyler, Skylor

Scott (English) from Scotland.
Scot, Scotto, Scotty

Scotty (English) a familiar form of Scott.
Scotie, Scotti, Scottie

Seamus (Irish) a form of James.
Seamas, Seumas

Sean (Hebrew) God is gracious. (Irish) a form of John.
Seaghan, Séan, Seán, Seanán, Seane, Seann, Shaan, Shane, Shaun, Shawn, Shon, Siôn

Sebastian (Greek) venerable. (Latin) revered.
Bastian, Sabastian, Sabastien, Sebastiano, Sebastien, Sébastien, Sebastin, Sebastion, Sebbie, Sebestyén, Sebo, Sepasetiano

Sebastien, Sébastien (French) forms of Sebastian.
Sebasten

Serge (Latin) attendant.
Seargeoh, Serg, Sergei, Sergio, Sergios, Sergius, Sergiusz, Serguel, Sirgio, Sirgios

Sergio (Italian) a form of Serge.
Serginio, Serigo, Serjio

Seth (Hebrew) appointed. Bible: the third son of Adam.
Set, Sethan, Sethe, Shet

Shad (Punjabi) happy-go-lucky.
Shadd

Shane (Irish) an alternate form of Sean.
Shaine, Shayn

Shannon (Irish) small and wise.
Shanan, Shannan, Shannen, Shanon

Sharif (Arabic) honest; noble.
Shareef, Sharef, Shareff, Shariff, Shariyf, Sharyif

Shaun (Irish) an alternate form of Sean.
Shaughan, Shaughn, Shauna, Shaunahan, Shaune, Shaunn

Shavar (Hebrew) comet.
Shavit

Shawn (Irish) an alternate form of Sean.
Shawen, Shawne, Shawnee, Shawnn, Shawon

Shayne (Irish) an alternate form of Sean.

Shea (Irish) courteous.
Shae, Shai, Shayan, Shaye, Shey

Shelby (English) ledge estate.
Shel, Shelbey, Shelbie, Shell, Shelley, Shelly

Sheldon (English) farm on the ledge.
Shel, Shelden, Sheldin, Shell, Shelley, Shelly, Shelton

Sherman (English) sheep shearer; resident of a shire.
Scherman, Schermann, Sherm, Shermann, Shermie, Shermy

Sidney (French) from Saint Denis, France.
Cydney, Sid, Sidnee, Sidon, Sidonio, Sydney, Sydny

Silas (Latin) forest dweller.
Si, Sias, Sylas

Simeon (French) a form of Simon.
Simone

Simon (Hebrew) he heard. Bible: in the Old Testament, the second son of Jacob and Leah; in the New Testament, one of the Twelve Disciples.
Saimon, Samien, Semon, Shimon, Si, Sim, Simao, Simen, Simeon, Simion, Simm, Simmon, Simmonds, Simmons, Simms, Simmy, Simonas, Simone, Simson, Simyon, Síomón, Symon, Szymon

Skylar (Dutch) an alternate form of Schuyler.
Skye, Skyelar

Skyler (Dutch) an alternate form of Schuyler.
Skye, Skyeler, Skylee

Solomon (Hebrew) peaceful. Bible: a king of Israel famous for his wisdom.
Salamen, Salamon, Salamun, Salaun, Salman, Salomo, Selim, Shelomah, Shlomo, Sol, Solamh, Solaman, Solly, Solmon, Soloman, Solomonas, Sulaiman

Sonny (English) a familiar form of Grayson, Madison.
Sonnie

Spencer (English) dispenser of provisions.
Spence, Spencre, Spenser

Spenser (English) an alternate form of Spencer. Literature: Edmund Spenser was the British poet who wrote *The Faerie Queene*.
Spanser, Spense

Stacey, Stacy (Greek) productive. (Latin) stable, calm.
Stace, Stacee

Stanley (English) stony meadow.
Stan, Stanlea, Stanlee, Stanleigh, Stanly

Stefan (German, Polish, Swedish) a form of Stephen.
Staffan, Staffon, Steafeán, Stefanson,

Stefaun, Stefawn, Steffan, Steffon

Stefano (Italian) a form of Stephen.

Steffen (Norwegian) a form of Stephen.
Stefen, Steffin, Stefin

Stephan (Greek) an alternate form of Stephen.
Stephanas, Stephano, Stephanos, Stephanus

Stephane (French) a ıorm of Stephen.
Stefane, Stepháne

Stephen (Greek) crowned. See also Esteban.
Stamos, Stavros, Stefan, Stefano, Stefanos, Stefen, Stenya, Stepan, Stepanos, Steph, Stephan, Stephanas, Stéphane, Stepháne, Stephano, Stephanos, Stephanus, Stephens, Stephenson, Stephfan, Stephin, Stephon, Stephone, Stepven, Steve, Steven, Stevie

Stephon (Greek) an alternate form of Stephen.
Stefon, Stefone, Stepfon, Stephone

Sterling (English) valuable; silver penny.

Steve (Greek) a short form of Stephen, Steven.
Steave, Steeve, Stevie, Stevy

Steven (Greek) crowned. An alternate form of Stephen.
Steevan, Steeven, Steiven, Stevan, Steve, Stevens, Stevie

Stevie (English) a familiar form of Stephen, Steven.
Stevey, Stevy

Stewart (English) an alternate form of Stuart.
Steward, Stu

Stuart (English) caretaker, steward. History: the Scottish and English royal dynasty.
Stewart, Stu, Stuarrt

Sundeep (Punjabi) light; enlightened.
Sundip

Syed (Arabic) happy.

Sylvain (French) a form of Sylvester.

Sylvester (Latin) forest dweller.
Silvester, Silvestro, Sly, Syl, Sylvain, Sylverster, Sylvestre

T

Tad (Greek, Latin) a short form of Thaddeus. (Welsh) father.
Tadd, Taddy, Tade, Tadek, Tadey

Tai (Vietnamese) weather; prosperous; talented.

Talon (French, English) claw, nail.
Tallin, Tallon

Tanner (English) leather worker, tanner.
Tan, Tanery, Tann, Tannor, Tanny

Tariq (Arabic) conqueror. History: Tarik was the Muslim general who conquered Spain.
Tareck, Tareek, Tarek, Tarick, Tarik, Tarreq, Tereik

Tate (Scandinavian, English) cheerful. (Native American) long-winded talker.
Tait, Tayte

Taurean (Latin) strong; forceful. Astrology: born under the sign of Taurus.
Tauris, Taurus

Tavaris (Aramaic) misfortune.
Tarvaris, Tarvarres, Tavar,
Tavaras, Tavares, Tavari,
Tavarian, Tavarius,
Tavarres, Tavarri, Tavarris,
Tavars, Tavarse, Tavarus,
Taveress, Tevaris, Tevarus

Taylor (English) tailor.
Tailer, Tailor, Talor, Tayler,
Taylour, Teyler

Ted (English) a short form
of Edward, Theodore.
Tedd, Tedek, Tedik,
Tedson

Teddy (English)
a familiar form of
Edward, Theodore.
Teddey, Teddie

Terell, Terrel (German)
alternate forms of Terrell.

Terence (Latin) an alternate
form of Terrence.
Teren, Teryn

Terrance (Latin) an alternate form of Terrence.
Tarrance, Tearance,
Tearrance, Terance,
Terran

Terrell (German) thunder
ruler.
Tarell, Terrail, Terral,
Terrale, Terrall, Terreal,
Terrelle, Terrill, Terryal,
Terryel, Tirel, Tirrell,
Turrell, Tyrel

Terrence (Latin) smooth.
Tarrance, Terence,
Terencio, Terrance,
Terren, Terry, Torrence,
Tyreese

Terry (English) a familiar
form of Terrence.
Tarry, Terrey, Terri, Terrie

Thaddeus (Greek) courageous. (Latin) praiser.
Bible: one of the Twelve
Apostles.
Tad, Taddeo, Taddeus,
Tadzio, Thad, Thaddaeus,
Thaddaus, Thaddeau,
Thaddeaus, Thaddeo,
Thaddiaus, Thaddius,
Thadeaou, Thadeous,
Thadeus, Thadieus,
Thadious, Thadius,
Thadus

Theo (English) a short form
of Theodore.

Theodore (Greek) gift
of God.
Téadóir, Teador, Ted,
Teddy, Tedor, Tedorek,
Telly, Teodomiro, Teodoro,
Teodus, Teos, Tewdor,
Theo, Theodor, Theódor,
Theodors, Theodorus,
Theodosios, Theodrekr,
Tivadar, Todor, Tolek,
Tudor

Theron (Greek) hunter.
Theran, Theren, Therin,
Therron

Thomas (Greek, Aramaic)
twin. Bible: one of the
Twelve Apostles.
**Tam, Tammy, Tavish,
Tevis, Thom, Thoma,
Thomason, Thomeson,
Thomison, Thompson,
Thomson, Tom, Toma,
Tomas, Tomasso, Tomcy,
Tomey, Tomi, Tomey,
Tommy, Toomas**

Tim (Greek) a short form
of Timothy.
Timmie, Timmy

Timmy (Greek) a familiar
form of Timothy.

Timothy (Greek) honoring
God.
**Tadhg, Taidgh, Tiege,
Tim, Tima, Timithy,
Timkin, Timmathy,
Timmothy, Timmoty,
Timmthy, Timmy, Timo,
Timofey, Timok, Timon,
Timontheo, Timonthy,
Timót, Timote, Timotei,
Timoteo, Timoteus,
Timothé, Timothée,
Timotheo, Timotheos,
Timotheus, Timothey,
Timthie, Tiomóid, Tisha,
Tomothy, Tymon,
Tymothy**

Titus (Greek) giant. (Latin)
hero. Bible: a recipient
of one of Paul's New
Testament letters.
Tite, Titek, Tito, Tytus

Tobias (Hebrew) God is
good.
**Tobia, Tobiah, Tobiás,
Tobin, Tobit, Toby, Tobyn,
Tovin, Tuvya**

Toby (Hebrew) a familiar
form of Tobias.
Tobby, Tobe, Tobey, Tobie

Todd (English) fox.
Tod, Toddie, Toddy

Tom (English) a short form
of Tomas, Thomas.
**Teo, Thom, Tommey,
Tommie, Tommy**

Tomas (German) a form
of Thomas.
**Tom, Tomaisin, Tomaz,
Tomcio, Tome, Tomek,
Tomelis, Tomico, Tomik,
Tomislaw, Tomo, Tomson**

Tommie (Hebrew) an alternate form of Tommy.
Tommi

Tommy (Hebrew) a familiar
form of Thomas.
Tommie

Tony (Greek) flourishing.
(Latin) praiseworthy.
(English) a short form of
Anthony.
**Tonda, Tonek, Toney,
Toni, Tonik, Tonio**

Torrence (Latin) an alter-
nate form of Terrence.
(Irish) knolls.
**Tawrence, Torance,
Toreence, Toren, Torin,
Torn, Torr, Torren,**

Torreon, Torrin, Torry, Tory, Tuarence, Turance

Torrey (English) an alternate form of Tory.
Toreey, Torre, Torri, Torrie, Torry

Tory (English) a familiar form of Torrence.
Tori, Torrey

Trace (Irish) an alternate form of Tracy.

Tracy (Greek) harvester. (Latin) courageous. (Irish) battler.
Trace, Tracey, Tracie, Treacy

Travis (English) crossroads.
Travais, Traves, Traveus, Travious, Traviss, Travus, Travys, Trevais

Tremaine, Tremayne (Scottish) house of stone.
Tramaine, Tremain, Treymaine, Trimaine

Trent (Latin) torrent, rapid stream. (French) thirty. Geography: a city in northern Italy.
Trente, Trentino, Trento, Trentonio

Trenton (Latin) town by the rapid stream. Geography: a city in New Jersey.
Trendon, Trendun, Trenten, Trentin, Trinton

Trevor (Irish) prudent. (Welsh) homestead.
Trefor, Trev, Trevar, Trever, Treyvor

Trey (English) three; third.
Trae, Trai, Tray

Tristan (Welsh) bold. Literature: a knight in the Arthurian legends who fell in love with his uncle's wife.
Trestan, Treston, Tris, Trisan, Tristano, Tristen, Tristian, Tristin, Triston, Trystan

Troy (Irish) foot soldier. (French) curly haired. (English) water.
Troi, Troye, Troyton

Tuan (Vietnamese) goes smoothly.

Tucker (English) fuller, tucker of cloth.
Tuck, Tuckie, Tucky

Ty (English) a short form of Tyler, Tyrone, Tyrus.
Tye

Tyler (English) tile maker.
Tiler, Ty, Tyel, Tylar, Tyle, Tylee, Tylere, Tyller, Tylor

Tylor (English) an alternate form of Tyler.

Tyree (Scottish) island dweller. Geography: Tiree is an island off the west coast of Scotland.
Tyra, Tyrae, Tyrai, Tyray, Tyre, Tyrea, Tyrée

Tyrel, Tyrell (American) forms of Terrell.

Tyrel, Tyrell (cont.)
Tyrelle, Tyrrel, Tyrrell

Tyron (American) a form
of Tyrone.
Tyronn, Tyronna, Tyronne

Tyrone (Greek) sovereign.
(Irish) land of Owen.
**Teirone, Terron, Ty,
Tyerone, Tyron, Tyroney,
Tyroon, Tyroun**

Tyson (French) son of Ty.
**Tison, Tiszon, Tyce, Tyesn,
Tyeson, Tysen, Tysie,
Tysne, Tysone**

U

Ulysses (Latin) wrathful.
**Ulick, Ulises, Ulishes,
Ulisse, Ulisses, Ulysse**

Uriah (Hebrew) my light.
Bible: the husband of
Bathsheba and a captain
in David's army.
**Uri, Uria, Urias,
Urijah, Yuri**

V

Van (Dutch) a short form
of Vandyke.
**Vander, Vane, Vann,
Vanno**

Vance (English) thresher.

Vandyke (Dutch) dyke.
Van

Vaughn (Welsh) small.
**Vaughan, Vaughen, Vaun,
Von, Voughn**

Vernon (Latin) springlike;
youthful.
**Vern, Vernen, Verney,
Vernin**

Vicente (Spanish) a form
of Vincent.
Vicent, Visente

Victor (Latin) victor,
conqueror.
**Vic, Victa, Victer,
Victoir, Victoriano,
Victorien, Victorin,
Victorio, Viktor, Vitin,
Vittorio, Wiktor**

Vijay (Hindi) victorious.
Religion: another name
for the Hindu god Shiva.

Vince (English) a short
form of Vincent.
Vence, Vint

W

Vincent (Latin) victor, conqueror.
Uinseann, Vencent, Vicente, Vicenzo, Vikent, Vikenti, Vikesha, Vin, Vince, Vincence, Vincens, Vincente, Vincentius, Vincents, Vincenty, Vincenzo, Vinci, Vinclen, Vincient, Vinciente, Vinny, Wincent

Vincenzo (Italian) a form of Vincent.
Vincenz, Vincenzio, Vinzenz

Virgil (Latin) rod bearer, staff bearer. Literature: a Roman poet best known for his epic *Aenid*.
Vergil, Virge, Virgial, Virgie, Virgilio

Vito (Italian) a form of Victor.
Veit, Vidal, Vital, Vitale, Vitalis, Vitas, Vitin, Vitis, Vitus, Vitya, Vytas

Vladimir (Russian) famous prince. See also Walter.
Vimka, Vlad, Vladamir, Vladik, Vladimar, Vladimeer, Vladimire, Vladjimir, Vladka, Vladko, Vladlen, Volodya, Volya, Vova, Wladimir

Wade (English) ford; river crossing.
Wadesworth, Wadie, Waide, Wayde, Waydell

Wallace (English) from Wales.
Wallach, Wallas, Wallie, Wallis, Wally, Walsh, Welsh

Walter (German) army ruler, general. (English) woodsman. See also Vladimir.
Valter, Vanda, Vova, Walder, Wally, Walt, Waltli, Walther, Waltr, Wat, Waterio, Watkins, Watson

Warren (German) general; warden; rabbit hutch.
Ware, Waring, Warrenson, Warrin, Warriner, Worrin

Waylon (English) land by the road.
Wallen, Walon, Way, Waylan, Wayland, Waylen, Waylin, Weylin

Wayne (English) wagon maker.

Wayne *(cont.)*
Wain, Wanye, Wayn,
Waynell, Wene

Wendell (German) wan-
derer. (English) good dale,
good valley.
Wandale, Wendall,
Wendel, Wendle, Wendy

Wesley (English) western
meadow.
Wes, Weslee, Wesleyan,
Weslie, Wesly, Wessley,
Westleigh, Westley

Westley (English) an alternate form of Wesley.

Weston (English) western
town.
West, Westen, Westin

Whitney (English) white
island; white water.
Whit, Whittney, Widney,
Widny

Wilbert (German) brilliant;
resolute.
Wilberto, Wilburt

Wilfred (German) deter-
mined peacemaker.
Wilferd, Wilfredo, Wilfrid,
Wilfride, Wilfried,
Wilfryd, Will, Willfred,
Willfried, Willie, Willy

Wilfredo (Spanish) a form
of Wilfred.
Fredo, Wifredo, Willfredo

Will (English) a short
form of William.
Wilm, Wim

Willard (German) deter-
mined and brave.

William (English) deter-
mined guardian. See also
Bill, Billy, Guillaume,
Guillermo, Liam.
Vasyl, Vilhelm, Vili,
Viliam, Viljo, Ville,
Villiam, Welfel, Wilek,
Wiliama, Wiliame,
Wiliame, Willaim, Willam,
Willeam, Willem,
Williams, Willil, Willis,
Williw, Willyam, Wim

Willie (German) a familiar
form of William.
Wile, Wille, Willey, Willi,
Willia, Willy, Wily

Willis (German) son of
Willie.
Willice, Wills, Willus

Wilson (English) son of
Will.
Wilkinson, Willson

Winston (English) friendly
town; victory town.
Win, Winsten, Winstonn,
Winton, Wynstan,
Wynston

Wyatt (French) little
warrior.
Wiatt, Wyat, Wyatte,
Wye, Wyeth

X

Xavier (Arabic) bright.
(Basque) owner of the
new house. See also Javier,
Salvatore.
**Xabier, Xaiver, Xaver,
Xavian, Xavon, Xever,
Xizavier, Xzaiver,
Xzavaier, Xzaver, Xzavier,
Xzavion, Zavier**

Y

Yakov (Russian) a form
of Jacob.
**Yaacob, Yaacov, Yaakov,
Yachov, Yacov, Yakob,
Yasha**

Yevgenyi (Russian) a form
of Eugene.
Gena, Yevgeni, Yevgenij

Yusuf (Arabic, Swahili)
a form of Joseph.
Yusef, Yusuff

Yves (French) young archer.
Ives, Yvens, Yvon

Z

Zacharia (Hebrew) an
alternate form of
Zachariah.
Zacaria

Zachariah (Hebrew) God
remembered.
**Zacarias, Zacarius, Zacary,
Zaccary, Zacharias,
Zachary, Zachory,
Zachury, Zako, Zaquero,
Zecharia, Zechariah,
Zecharya, Zeggery, Zeke,
Zhachory**

Zacharie (Hebrew)
an alternate form of
Zachary.
Zachare, Zacharee

Zachary (Hebrew) God
remembered. A familiar
form of Zachariah.
History: Zachary Taylor
was the twelfth U.S.
president.
**Zacary, Zaccary,
Zach, Zacha, Zachaios,
Zacharey, Zachari,
Zacharia, Zacharias,
Zacharie, Zachaury,
Zachery, Zachry, Zack,
Zackary, Zackery,
Zakary, Zeke**

Zachery (Hebrew) an alternate form of Zachary.
Zacherey, Zacheria,
Zacherias, Zacheriah,
Zacherie, Zacherius

Zackary (Hebrew) an alternate form of Zachary.
Zack, Zackari, Zacharia,
Zackariah, Zackarie,
Zackery, Zackie, Zackorie,
Zackory, Zackree,
Zackrey, Zackry

Zackery (Hebrew) an alternate form of Zachery.

Zane (English) a form of John.
Zain, Zayne

Zechariah (Hebrew) an alternate form of Zachariah.
Zecharia, Zekarias, Zeke,
Zekeriah

Worksheets

Baby Name Worksheet

Mom's Favorite Names

rating	girls' names	rating	boys' names

Baby Name Worksheet
Dad's Favorite Names

rating	girls' names	rating	boys' names

Also from Meadowbrook Press

✦ **The Best Baby Shower Book**
The number one baby shower planner has been updated for the new millennium. This contemporary guide for planning baby showers is full of helpful hints, recipes, decorating ideas, and activities that are fun without being juvenile.

✦ **First-Year Baby Care**
This is one of the leading baby-care books to guide you through your baby's first year with complete information on the basics of baby care, including bathing, diapering, medical facts, and feeding your baby. Includes step-by-step illustrated instructions to make finding information easy, newborn screening and immunization schedules, breastfeeding information for working mothers, expanded information on child care options, reference guides to common illnesses, and environmental and safety tips.

✦ **Pregnancy, Childbirth, and the Newborn - Revised**
More complete and up-to-date than any other pregnancy guide, this remarkable book is the "bible" for childbirth educators. Now revised with a greatly expanded treatment of pregnancy tests, complications, and infections; an expanded list of drugs and medications (plus advice for uses); and a brand-new chapter on creating a detailed birth plan.